Frozen Section Library

Series Editor
Philip T. Cagle, MD
Houston, Texas, USA

For further volumes:
http://www.springer.com/series/7869

Frozen Section Library: Breast

by

Syed K. Mohsin

Department of Pathology, Riverside Methodist Hospital, Columbus, OH, USA

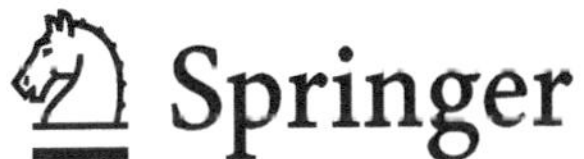

Syed K. Mohsin, MD
Department of Pathology
Riverside Methodist Hospital
Columbus, OH, USA
smohsin@ohiohealth.com

ISSN 1868-4157 e-ISSN 1868-4165
ISBN 978-1-4614-0717-1 ISBN 978-1-4614-0718-8 (eBook)
DOI 10.1007/978-1-4614-0718-8
Springer New York Dordrecht Heidelberg London

Library of Congress Control Number: 2011935991

Printed on acid-free paper

Springer is part of Springer Science+Business Media (www.springer.com)

To my wife, Hena, and to Leya, Bilal, and Alisha
Syed K. Mohsin

Series Preface

For over 100 years, the frozen section has been utilized as a tool for the rapid diagnosis of specimens while a patient is undergoing surgery, usually under general anesthesia, as a basis for making immediate treatment decisions. Frozen section diagnosis is often a challenge for the pathologist who must render a diagnosis that has crucial import for the patient in a minimal amount of time. In addition to the need for rapid recall of differential diagnoses, there are many pitfalls and artifacts that add to the risk of frozen section diagnosis that are not present with permanent sections of fully processed tissues that can be examined in a more leisurely fashion. Despite the century-long utilization of frozen sections, most standard pathology textbooks, both general and subspecialty, largely ignore the topic of frozen sections. Few textbooks have ever focused exclusively on frozen section diagnosis and those textbooks that have done so are now out-of-date and have limited illustrations.

Frozen Section Library Series is meant to provide convenient, user-friendly handbooks for each organ system to expedite use in the rushed frozen section situation. These books are small and lightweight, copiously color illustrated with images of actual frozen sections, highlighting pitfalls, artifacts, and differential diagnosis. The advantages of a series of organ-specific handbooks, in addition to the ease-of-use and manageable size, are that (1) a series allows more comprehensive coverage of more diagnoses, both common and rare, than a single volume that tries to highlight a limited number of diagnoses for each organ and (2) a series allows more detailed insight by permitting experienced authorities to emphasize the peculiarities of frozen section for each organ system.

As a handbook for practicing pathologists, these books are indispensable aids to diagnosis and avoiding dangers in one of the most challenging situations that pathologists encounter. Rapid consideration of differential diagnoses and how to avoid traps caused by frozen section artifacts are emphasized in these handbooks. A series of concise, easy-to-use, well-illustrated handbooks alleviates the often frustrating and time-consuming, sometimes futile, process of searching through bulky textbooks that are unlikely to illustrate or discuss pathologic diagnoses from the perspective of frozen sections in the first place. Tables and charts provide guidance for differential diagnosis of various histologic patterns. Touch preparations, which are used for some organs such as central nervous system or thyroid more often than others, are appropriately emphasized and illustrated according to the need for each specific organ.

This series is meant to benefit practicing surgical pathologists, both community and academic, and to pathology residents and fellows; and also to provide valuable perspectives to surgeons, surgery residents, and fellows who must rely on frozen section diagnosis by their pathologists. Most of all, we hope that this series contributes to the improved care of patients who rely on the frozen section to help guide their treatment.

Philip T. Cagle, MD

Preface

The use of intraoperative evaluation of breast specimens has evolved over the years. This evolution has seen the days with answering the typical questions asked by the surgeons for any oncologic surgery, i.e., diagnosis of a mass lesion, evaluation of margins, lymph node status, etc. In the past, some special handing requests such as harvesting fresh tissue for biochemical hormone receptors were quite unique to breast tumors. In the current practice, most surgical pathology suites and frozen section laboratories spend considerable amounts of time dealing with breast specimens, which is the result of rising volume of breast specimens in part related to improved screening for breast cancer and more well-educated patients.

Frozen Section Library on Breast is written with the intention of providing a handy reference book on topics covered only in piecemeal fashion in textbooks dedicated to breast pathology. In the current practice, the most important intraoperative evaluation is the examination of sentinel lymph nodes for breast cancer, and the techniques used for their evaluation are discussed in detail. The difficulties associated with frozen section for other intraoperative questions, such as margin evaluation, diagnosis, are covered in the subsequent chapters. The protocols for gross examination of breast specimens with a mass or nonpalpable lesion are provided. Finally, the changes in tissue fixation and handling for specimens to be used for predictive factors and their effects on workflow and standard operating procedure of grossing areas in anatomic pathology are discussed, covering activities performed in the gross room dealing with all types of breast specimens.

This handbook is targeted to pathologists, both in academics and private practice, residents, fellows, and pathology assistants. For this reason, I had help and input from my assistants, Bing,

Michelle, Allison, and Erica, to whom I am greatly indebted. This work is also intended to serve as a handy reference to other trainees rotating in Pathology Department about the nuances of adequately handling breast specimens in a fashion that meets the increasingly complex environment of breast pathology. It is hoped that this work adds to current body of literature in breast pathology in general, and provides a unique and much needed reference in particular.

Columbus, OH Syed K. Mohsin, MD

Contents

Chapter 1
Sentinel Lymph Nodes

One of the most important prognostic factors in breast cancer is the involvement of regional lymph nodes. Until recently, axillary lymph node dissection was the standard of care in the primary surgical management of breast cancer. However, it has been replaced with sentinel lymph node biopsy or dissection (SLND). Several studies have shown that SLND identifies the most likely involved lymph nodes, in fact accurately reflecting the status of axillary lymph nodes in over 90% of the cases. In addition, clinical trials have demonstrated that patients who undergo SLND are less likely to suffer from complications, such as lymphedema, neuropathy and other functional deficiencies and often do not require hospital stay, thus reducing cost and anxiety. The current practice is to perform SLND in all breast cancer patients with clinically negative axilla. If sentinel nodes are positive, then the patients are offered a completion axillary clearing.

About 25–30% of patients undergoing SLND are found to have positive nodes, requiring full axillary dissection. In order to prevent a second surgical procedure, the patients are consented to get SLND with intraoperative evaluation and if positive, to finish axillary clearance in the same surgical procedure. A coordinated effort between the breast surgeon and the pathologist can lead to highly accurate assessment of the sentinel lymph nodes (SLN) during the surgical procedure. The practice and protocols for intraoperative evaluation of SLND specimens vary among institutions. The two most common methods include frozen section (FS) and touch imprint cytology (TIC). There are a few molecular methods to detect metastases in SLN; however, they are not widely adopted. More recently, rapid immunohistochemical staining methods

S.K. Mohsin, *Frozen Section Library: Breast*, Frozen Section Library 9,
DOI 10.1007/978-1-4614-0718-8_1,

have also been developed as an aide to these two methods. This chapter mainly focuses on the first two techniques, which have been widely used and there is a large body of literature describing the pros and cons of these two methods. A brief overview of the molecular techniques is also provided.

IDENTIFICATION OF THE SLN

The technique of identification of the SLN is fairly well established. At most centers, a combination of radioisotope and blue dye is employed with or without preoperative lymphoscintigraphy. Technitium 99 sulfur colloid is injected intradermally above the tumor or peritumorally or around the areola. Some surgeons prefer to inject at the previous biopsy site. The amount of the radiotracer given to the patient varies depending upon the time interval between the injection and the actual procedure of SLN identification. About 300 mCi is an average dose for the same day procedure. A higher dose up to 500 mCi can be used for the next day procedure. Either isosulfan blue or methylene blue is used just before the procedure to increase the probability of a successful SLN identification procedure. A handheld gamma counter is used to measure radioactivity. A SLN is defined as a blue lymph node and/or a node with radioactive count above the baseline. The process is continued to keep looking for lymph nodes until the counts are ≤10% of the maximal. The SLN are labeled as hot and blue or blue only or hot only, followed by the radioactive count. The surgical technique of dissection of the SLN is variable. Some surgeons like to remove the surrounding fat and provide a discrete lymph node, while others tend to find as many nodes in the area of radioactivity and remove the nodes together with surrounding adipose tissue.

GROSSING TECHNIQUE

After appropriate identification of the specimen containers and the accompanying requisition, tissue should be carefully dissected using visual and palpation method to identify all the lymph nodes in the specimen. After counting the lymph nodes, each should be measured in three dimensions and described paying attention to the appearance (Fig. 1.1). It is preferable to remove as much fat around the lymph node as possible to make the next steps easier. SLN should then be carefully sliced using new, sharp blade at 2-mm intervals, as per guidelines from the College of American Pathologists (CAP). It is at the discretion of the pathologist whether to use short or long axis of the node for slicing. However, the idea is to try to examine as large a cut surface as possible during the intraoperative and permanent

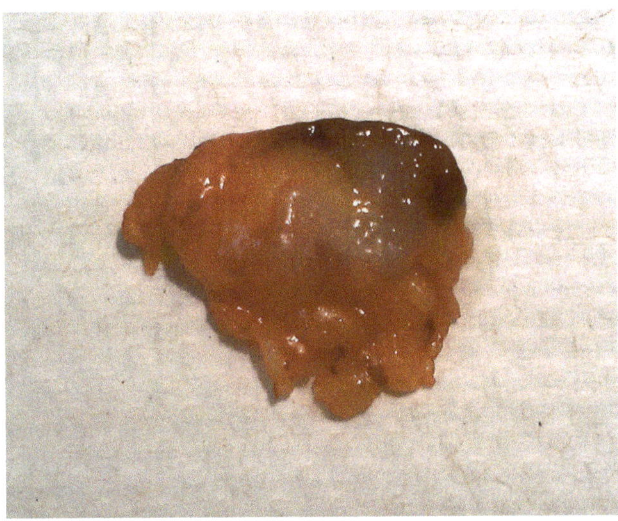

FIGURE 1.1 Gross appearance of a SLN. This small node shows blue dye in the subcapsular sinus and some attached adipose tissue on the inferior aspect.

section assessment. Theoretically, slicing the node in the short axis may be more useful to achieve this objective.

PREPARATION OF SLIDES FOR MICROSCOPIC EXAMINATION

The methods and exact protocols for microscopic assessment of SLN, including both the intraoperative and final examination, are variable and more than 100 variations have been reported in the literature. This chapter focuses primarily on the intraoperative assessment. In general, it is up to the individual laboratory and in some institutions, the discretion of the pathologist to use FS and/or TIC. If both the techniques are used, then the touch imprints are prepared before FS. Slides should be labeled with patient's name and specimen identification, such as "SLN A" or "SLN #1." An appropriate amount of OCT compound should be used to aid in preparing FS. If more than one slice of a SLN is placed in one FS block, then creating a solid base of OCT compound is recommended to help place all the tissue pieces in one plane. This helps prevent loss of tissue during trimming into the OCT block. A few extra seconds spent to trim the fat around the SLN is worth for obtaining a good FS.

FROZEN SECTION PREPARATION

FS is the most commonly employed method for intraoperative examination of SLN, reported by as many as 75% of the laboratories. This is true despite some of the known limitations of this technique. There is significant variation among the laboratories regarding the technique and the protocol of FS for SLN. Some laboratories use either isopentane baths or liquid nitrogen, while the others employ cooling bars or heat extractors to freeze the tissue. The first two methods provide rapid cooling to –45 to –70°C temperature, decreasing the chances of ice crystal formation but can cause freeze cracks in the tissue. On the other hand, tissue frozen in the cryostat using heat extractors or freezing bars is more prone to ice crystal formation that can affect morphology but allows for easier frozen section microtomy. The number of H&E sections examined and the amount of trimming in between these levels can also affect sensitivity, specificity and accuracy of FS in SLN. The use of hematoxylin and eosin staining is fairly standard in FS methodology. For pathologic assessment of SLN either by FS or TIC, *sensitivity* is defined as the percentage of positive intraoperative cases among those with positive permanent section pathology. *Specificity* is defined as the percentage of negative intraoperative results among those cases with negative permanent section pathology. In most studies, the positive results on the permanent section histology include isolated tumor cells (ITC), micrometastases and macrometastases. *ITC* are defined as small clusters of cells not greater than 0.2 mm in largest dimension, or single cells, usually with little if any histologic stromal reaction. They may be detected by routine histology or by immunohistochemical or molecular methods. *Micrometastases* are defined as tumor deposits greater than 0.2 mm but not more than 2.0 mm in largest dimension. All metastases greater than 2.0 mm are classified as macrometases or simply metastases.

FS EVALUATION OF SLN

There are certain advantages in interpreting FS of SLN. The most important is the ability to assess morphologic features of the tumor. A quick overview on low power focused initially on the subcapsular sinus should identify most of the metastasis. FS also provides an opportunity to measure the size of the metastasis. In certain cases, this can be a very valuable piece of information to the surgeon, particularly in light of recent results of a clinical trial, which showed that it might be reasonable to forego full axillary dissection in patients with limited or small metastasis in SLN without necessarily compromising long-term survival.

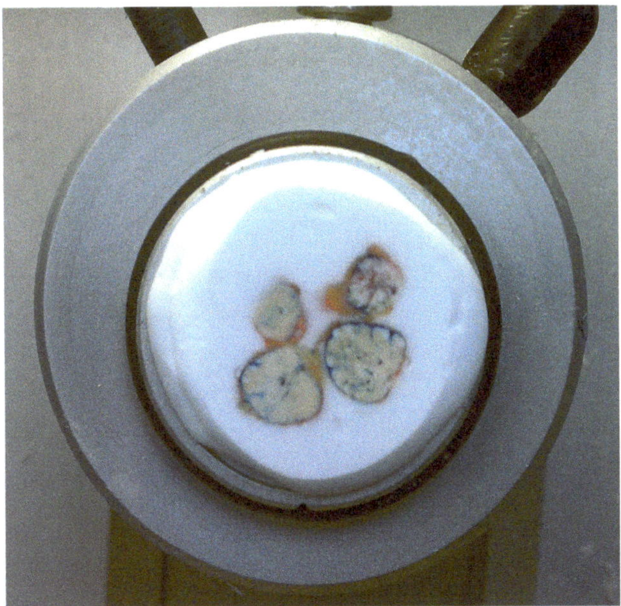

FIGURE 1.2 Examination of trimmed frozen section block in the cryostat. One of the helpful steps during the intraoperative assessment of SLN is to review the node as it seen here. Note the *blue dye* in the subcapsular sinuses and nodular appearance of the node. This is the typical appearance of a reactive lymph node.

The microscopic evaluation of the FS from SLN is relatively straightforward. One of the first steps is to examine the trimmed OCT block in the cryostat (Figs. 1.2 and 1.3). This can highlight the overall architecture of the lymph node and often shows the tumor as pale gray–white areas or nodules. The normal or reactive lymphoid tissue appears tan or fish flesh like while fat is bright yellow. Initially, the entire histologic section should be examined at low power to look for obvious metastatic tumor (Figs. 1.4 and 1.5). Then the subcapsular sinus of the lymph node should be screened at an intermediate magnification, as this is the most common site of involvement by metastatic carcinoma. Care should be taken not to miss very small clusters of epithelial cells. Then the rest of the node can be examined (Figs. 1.6–1.21). Sinus histiocytes and some blood vessels with prominent endothelial cells can be mimic small clusters of epithelial cells. Usually a comparison of such worrisome cells with other areas of the lymph node provides a good reference to resolve the differential diagnosis (Table 1.1 and Figs. 1.22–1.24).

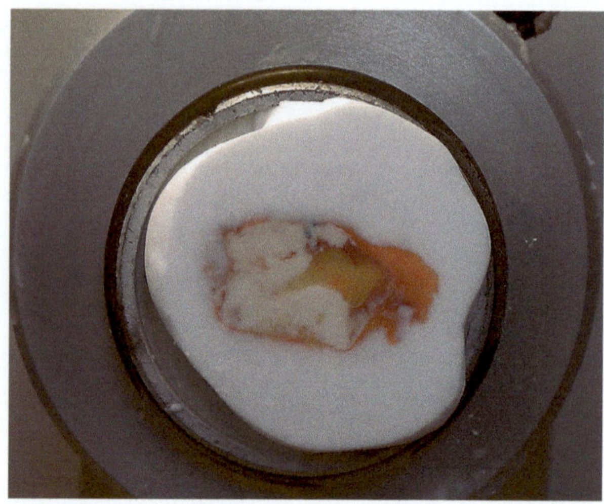

FIGURE 1.3 Frozen section block of a positive SLN. In this case, the SLN architecture is distorted. The cortex looks expanded and *pale white* and *blue dye* is difficult to identify. This can be a clue to expect metastatic tumor in the frozen section slide.

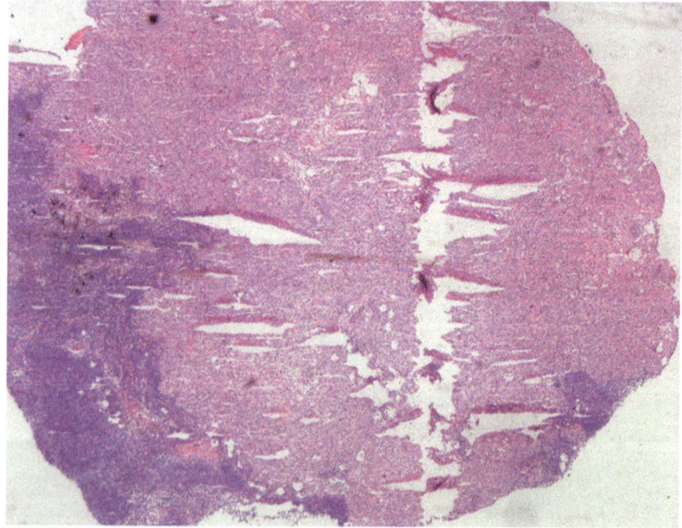

FIGURE 1.4 Frozen section of a positive SLN. This case is straightforward to interpret. Most of the node is replaced by metastatic carcinoma.

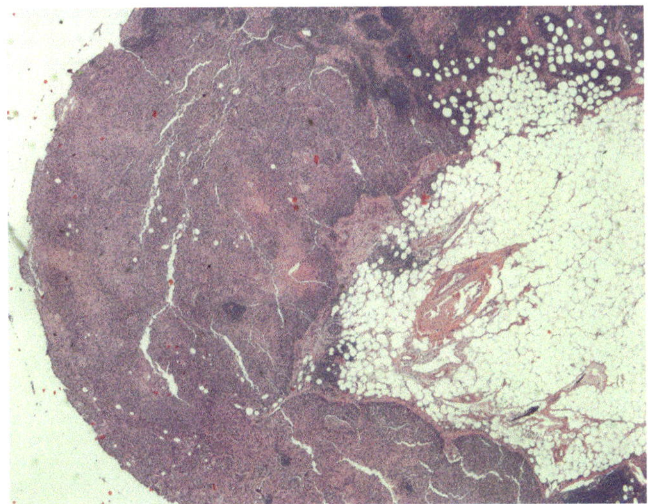

FIGURE 1.5 Permanent section of a SLN positive on frozen section. In this case, the frozen section (not shown) contained metastatic cells but due to fat in the middle of the node, the size of metastasis could not be accurately measured.

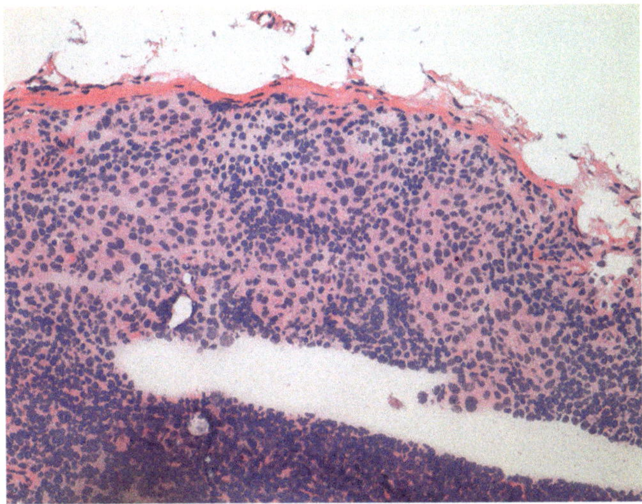

FIGURE 1.6 Frozen section of a positive SLN with air-drying artifact. The subcapsular sinus contains several clusters of cells with moderate amount of cytoplasm. However, there is some air-drying artifact, which makes it difficult to interpret these cells.

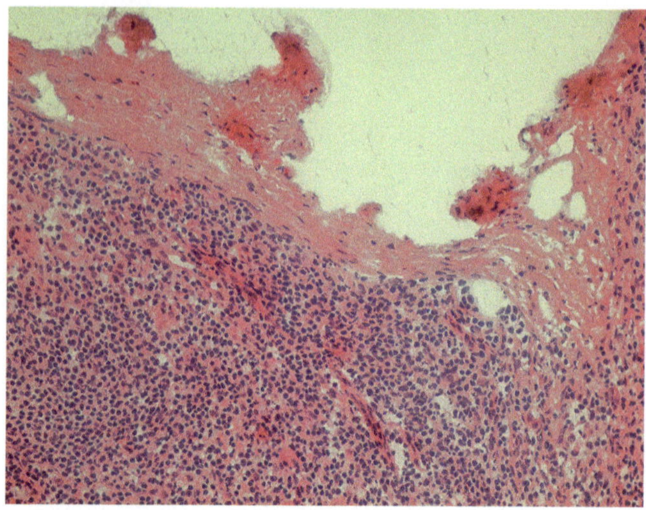

FIGURE 1.7 Frozen section of a false negative SLN for micrometastasis. In this case, no metastatic tumor is seen in the frozen section. However, the final pathology showed micrometastasis.

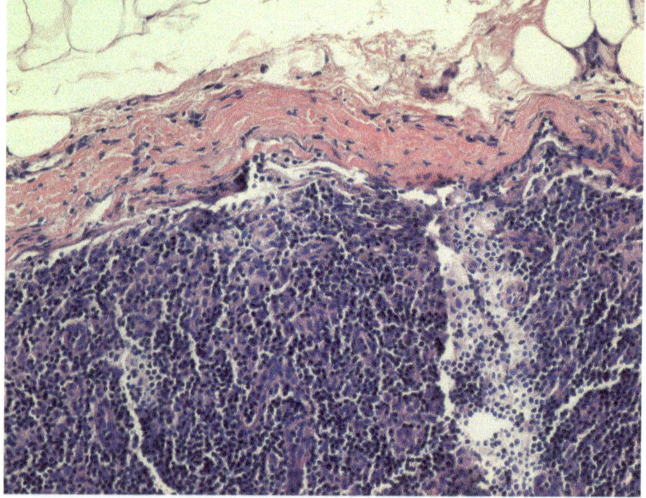

FIGURE 1.8 Permanent section of the false negative SLN seen in Fig. 1.7. No definite metastatic cells are identified in this section. The final pathology showed micrometastasis (see Fig. 1.9).

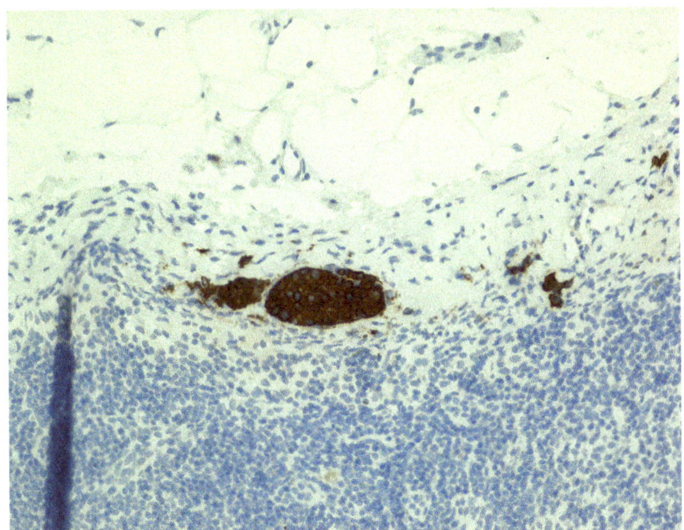

FIGURE 1.9 Cytokeratin immunostain on SLN seen in Figs. 1.7 and 1.8. The subcapsular sinus contains keratin-positive clusters and a few single cells, consistent with micrometastasis.

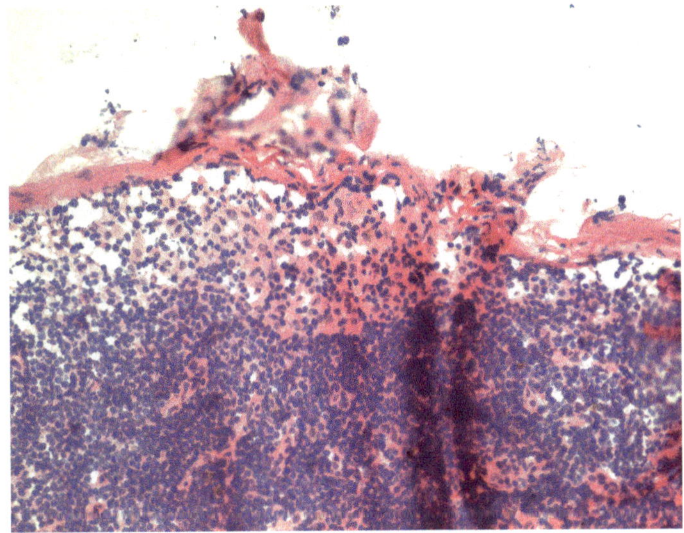

FIGURE 1.10 Frozen section of a false negative SLN. This reasonable frozen section of the SLN failed to detect ITC or metastases.

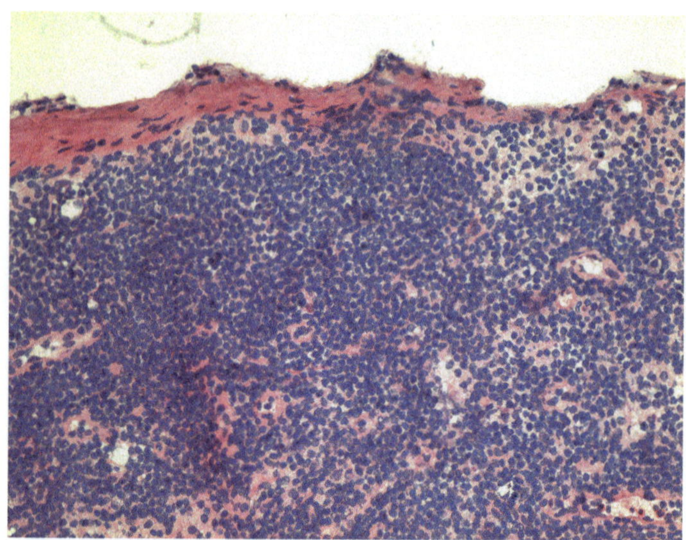

FIGURE 1.11 Permanent section of the false negative SLN seen in Fig. 1.10. In this case, no ITC or micrometastasis is identified on the slide.

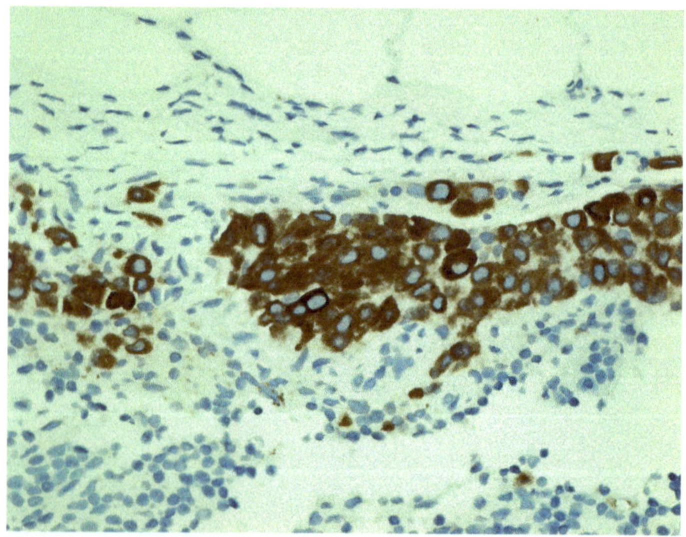

FIGURE 1.12 Cytokeratin immunostain on SLN seen in Figs. 1.10 and 1.11. There are small sheets and confluent metastatic cells, consistent with micrometastasis.

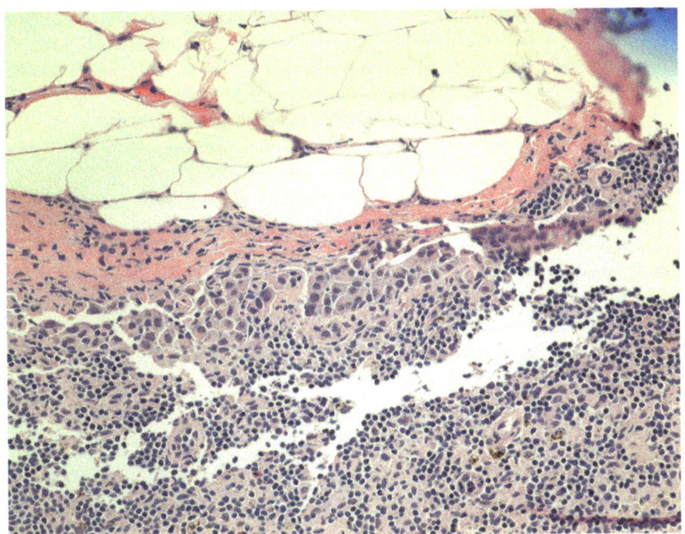

FIGURE 1.13 High power view of frozen section of SLN. A few clusters of metastatic carcinoma cells are identified in the subcapsular sinus.

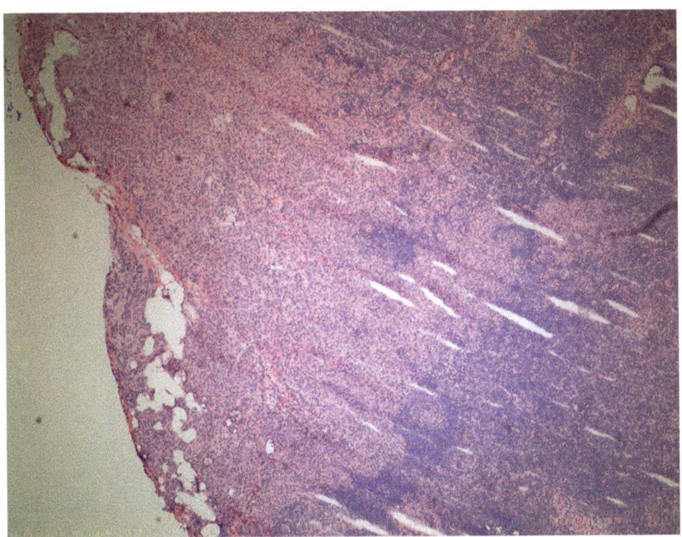

FIGURE 1.14 Another example of frozen section of a positive SLN. This node shows obvious metastatic disease.

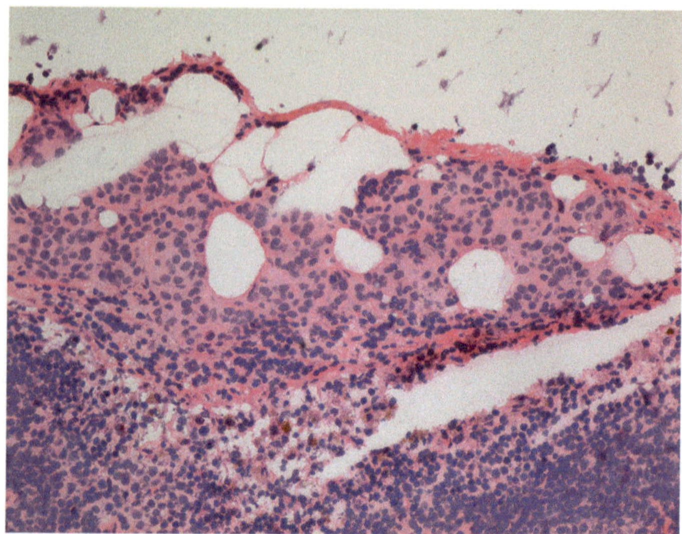

FIGURE 1.15 Frozen section of a positive SLN. This FS not only shows the metastatic carcinoma, but it also demonstrates some tumor nests in adipose tissue, raising the possibility of extranodal extension of the tumor.

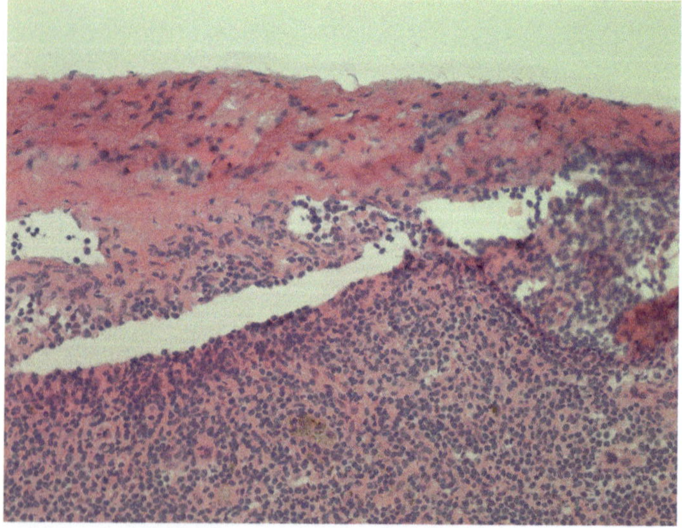

FIGURE 1.16 Frozen section of a false negative SLN for ITC. The quality is good to evaluate the subcapsular sinus and it is negative for metastatic cells.

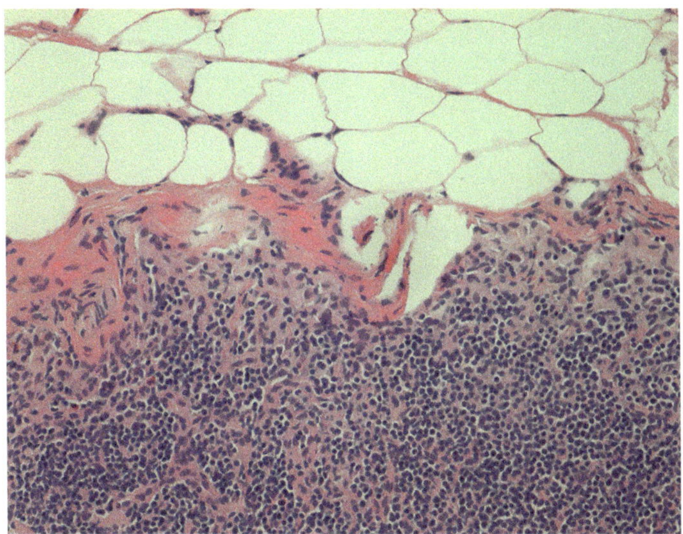

FIGURE 1.17 Permanent section of the SLN from Fig. 1.16. Even this higher quality H&E slide fails to show ITC.

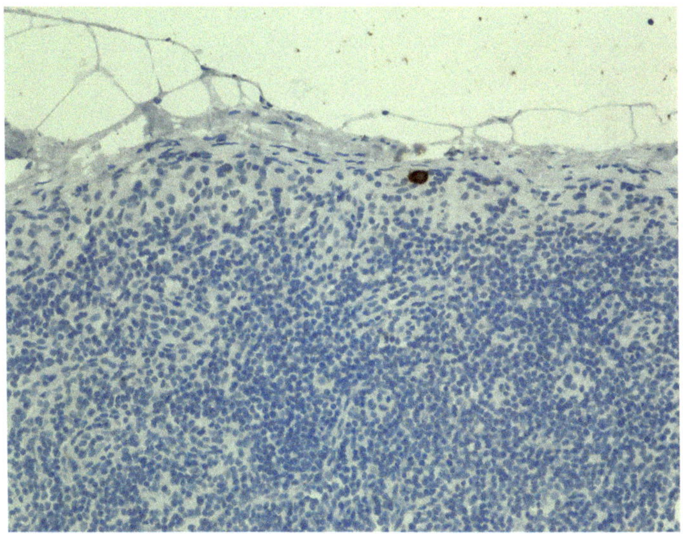

FIGURE 1.18 Cytokeratin immunostain on the SLN from Figs. 1.16 and 1.17. This shows a single positive cell in the subcapsular sinus. This is the minimal requirement for the diagnosis of ITC.

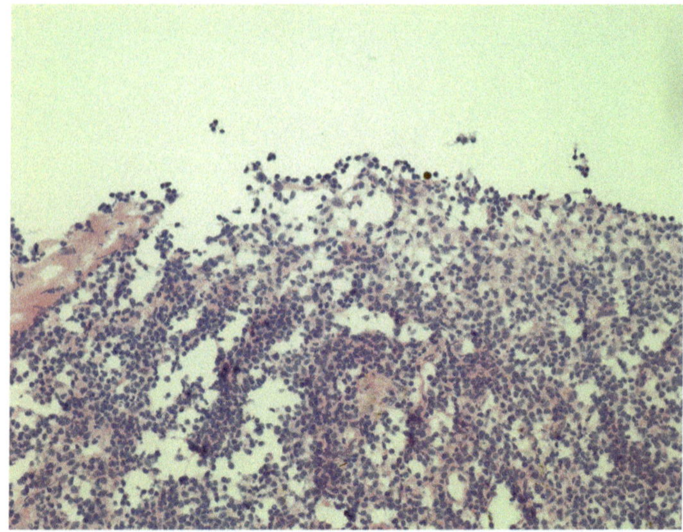

FIGURE 1.19 Frozen section of a false negative SLN. The capsule is disrupted and the evaluation of the subcapsular sinus is less than optimal. The possibility of isolated tumor cells and micrometastasis cannot be ruled out.

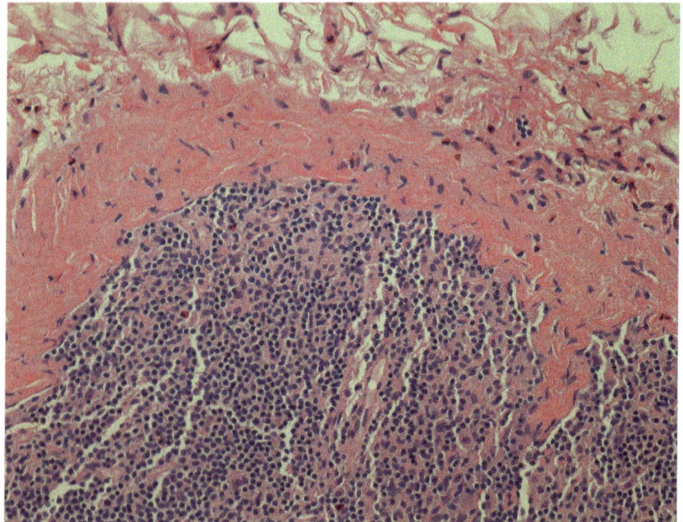

FIGURE 1.20 Permanent section of the SLN from Fig. 1.19. ITC by definition cannot be seen on prospective review of H&E stained sections.

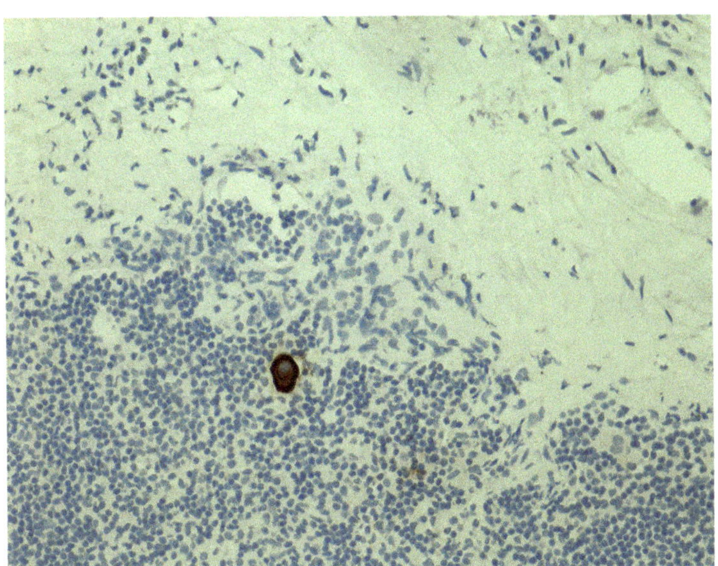

FIGURE 1.21 Cytokeratin immunostain on the SLN from Figs. 1.19 and 1.20. This case shows a single cytokeratin-positive ITC in the lymph node. In this section, the cell appears to be just below the subcapsular sinus.

TABLE 1.1 Key steps during microscopic assessment of FS of SLN.

- The information about the primary tumor, such as histologic type and grade should be available to the pathologist prior to evaluating the SLN
- Scan the section at low power to rule out large metastasis
- Use intermediate magnification to look for micrometastasis, focusing on subcapsular sinus
- Use higher magnification to confirm small clusters of metastatic cells or try to identify rare tumor cells
- Once the metastatic tumor cells are identified, it should be correlated with the histologic features of the primary tumor
- Sinus histiocytes can mimic metastasis. A comparison with cells in other areas of the lymph node is helpful
- Metastatic cells often have more dense and discrete cytoplasm than histiocytes

There are certain limitations and pitfalls of FS of SLN. These include irreversible loss of valuable tissue during the trimming process by as much as 50% in some studies, false negative result due to incomplete sectioning or inadequate levels examined,

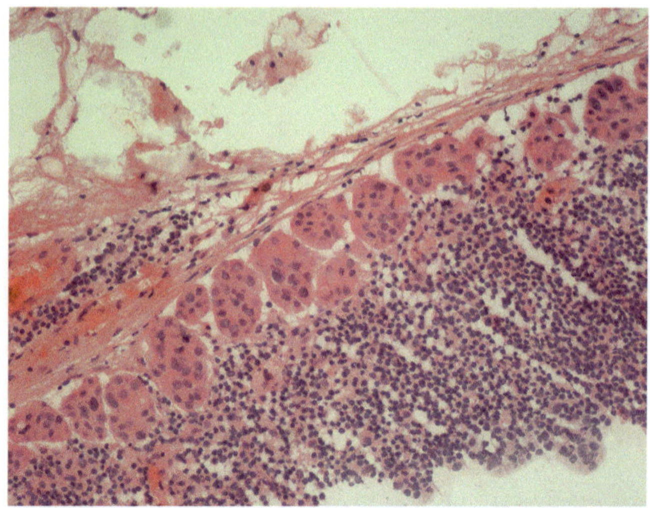

FIGURE 1.22 Frozen section of a SLN positive for micropapillary carcinoma. This type of invasive carcinoma has a higher propensity to involve the lymph nodes. A prior knowledge of this diagnosis is helpful to the pathologist performing intraoperative assessment of SLN to look for small metastases.

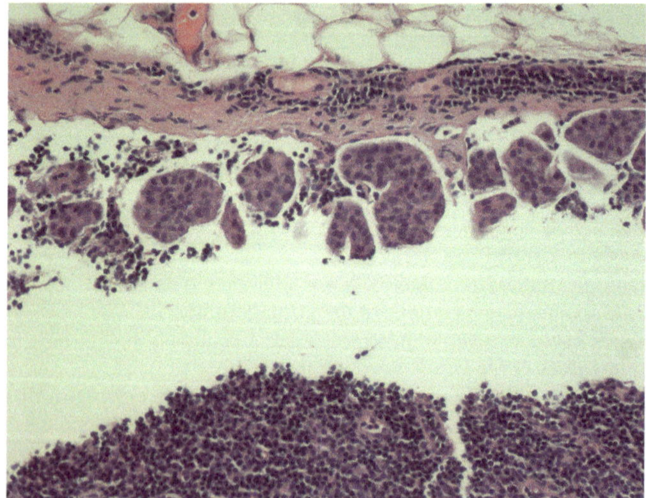

FIGURE 1.23 Permanent section of the positive SLN seen in Fig. 1.22. There is a processing artifact, where micropapillary carcinoma in the sinus is separated from the rest of the lymph node.

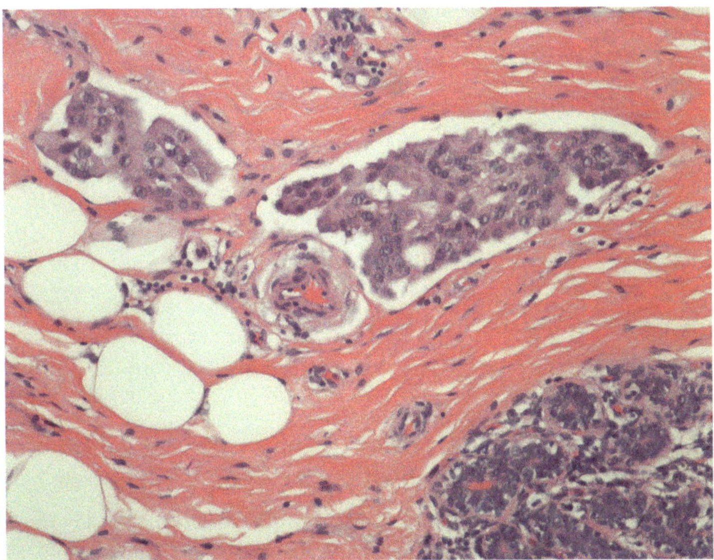

FIGURE 1.24 Lymphovascular invasion in the primary micropapillary carcinoma seen in Figs. 1.22 and 1.23. Tumor is present in the lymphatic channels next to a normal breast epithelial unit.

higher cost of the procedure as compared to TIC, longer time needed to prepare and stain the sections and rare false positive result mainly due to artifacts introduced during the freezing or sectioning of inadequately frozen tissue. Some of these concerns have been addressed in several studies and have been used as arguments against the use of FS for SLN. In fact, some studies that have performed exhaustive search by examining serial sections of the entire SLN to exhaustion of tissue block report that metastatic tumor may continue to be discovered throughout the lymph node (Figs. 1.25 and 1.26). Whether such small metastatic tumor deposits are of clinical significance or not can be argued. The current American Joint Committee on Cancer (AJCC) guidelines for breast cancer staging do address this issue by separating ITC as node-negative disease as compared to micrometastasis and macrometastases as node-positive disease. The success of FS in identifying such small metastatic deposits depends on expertise of the technician preparing FS, staining quality, the amount of fat around and within the lymph node and the time spent by the pathologist examining the sections (Figs. 1.27 and 1.28). In studies

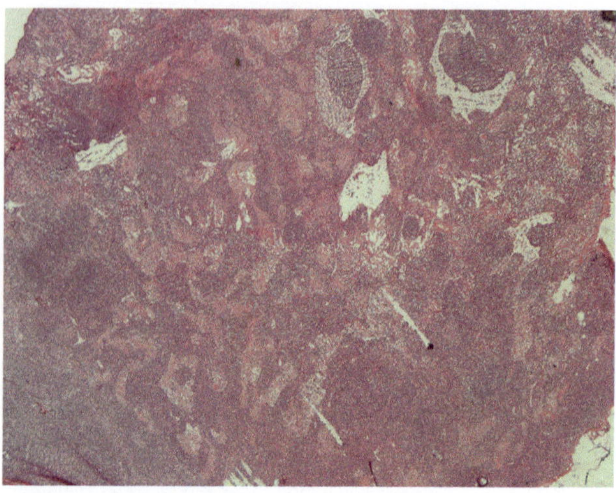

FIGURE 1.25 Excessive trimming of SLN during FS. Intact and fully faced SLN before trimming for frozen section. One of the major disadvantages of frozen section of SLN is irreversible loss of tissue. See Fig. 1.26 for the result of aggressive trimming of the tissue during frozen section.

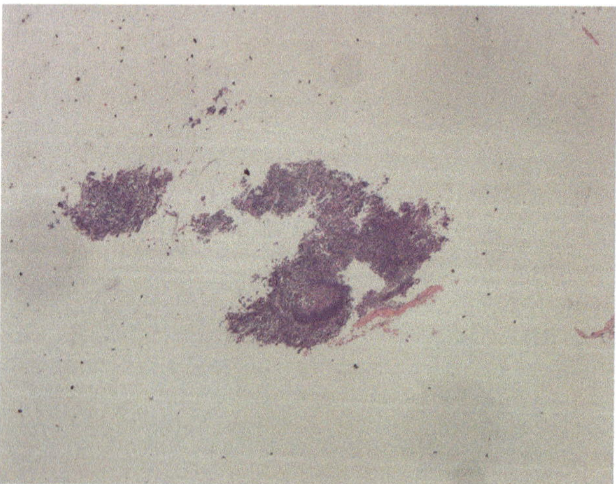

FIGURE 1.26 Permanent section of the overtrimmed SLN seen in Fig. 1.25. There is a substantial loss of nodal tissue from this SLN due to excessive trimming of the frozen section block. Most of the tissue was cut off, leaving minimal material for permanent section evaluation.

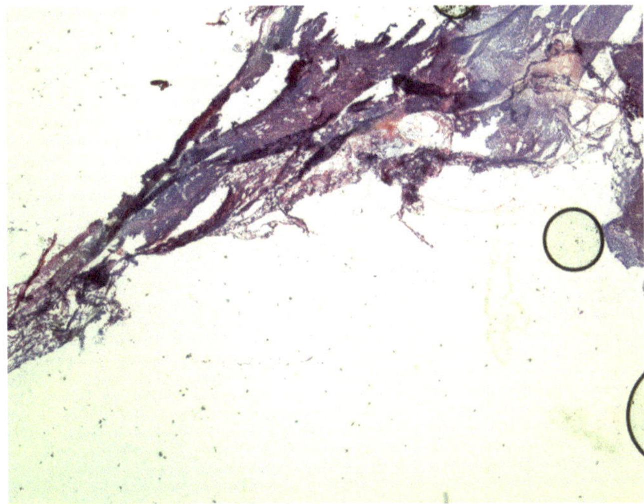

FIGURE 1.27 Poor quality of frozen section missed metastasis in a SLN. This frozen section was poorly cut and failed to get a full face of the tissue. This can be due to lack of experience of the histotechnologist, who is trying to preserve the tissue or poor technique of freezing and cutting frozen section. There are folds in the tissue and obvious missing pieces.

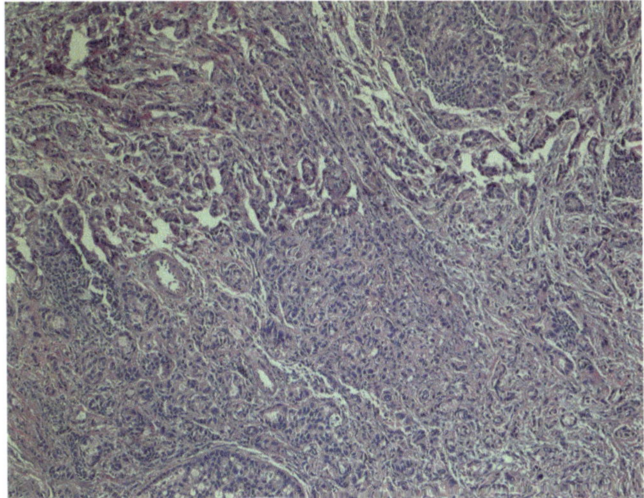

FIGURE 1.28 Permanent section of the SLN shown in Fig. 1.27. There is an obvious metastatic tumor in this node. Note some freeze artifact as well.

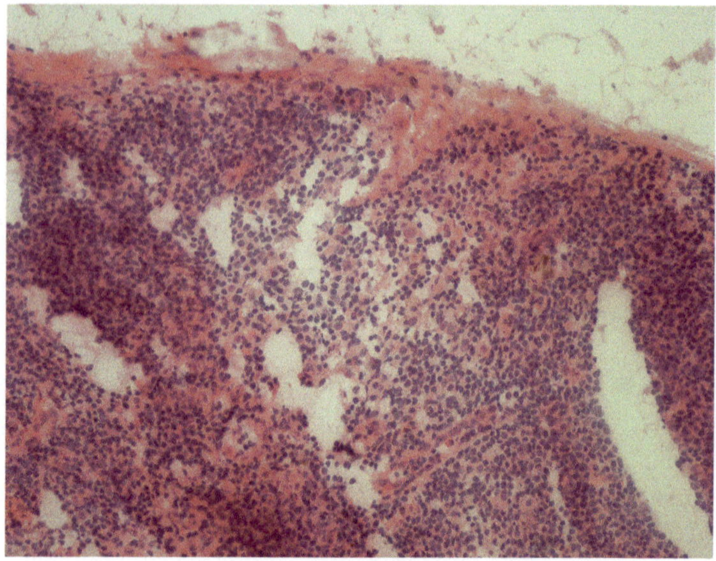

FIGURE 1.29 Frozen section of SLN subsequently found to have ITC. The section is of reasonable quality, but no definite epithelial cells are identified. This is a major limitation of frozen section for SLN and is associated with very low sensitivity.

examining the potential causes of low accuracy of FS, a large number of discordance has been related to the small size of the metastatic tumor (<2 mm), and accuracy as low as 15% has been reported in this subgroup (Figs. 1.29 and 1.30). An additional limitation of the FS is identification of low nuclear grade metastatic tumors and particularly lobular carcinomas. Some of the studies looking specifically at these numbers in lobular carcinoma are summarized in Table 1.2.

However, the degree of concordance and its measures such as sensitivity, specificity and accuracy depend on a variety of factors involved in the intraoperative as well as permanent section histopathologic evaluation. Some of the protocols used for grossing SLN include serial sectioning of SLN at 1.5–2 mm intervals irrespective of the size of the node versus bisecting the SLN if more than 3 or 5 or even 10 mm in size. There is also tremendous variation in the way and the number of sections examined during FS, e.g., single H&E level, 2 or 3 levels from each half or pieces, serial sections versus step levels with the interval between each level ranging from 50 to 250 microns. There are also a number of

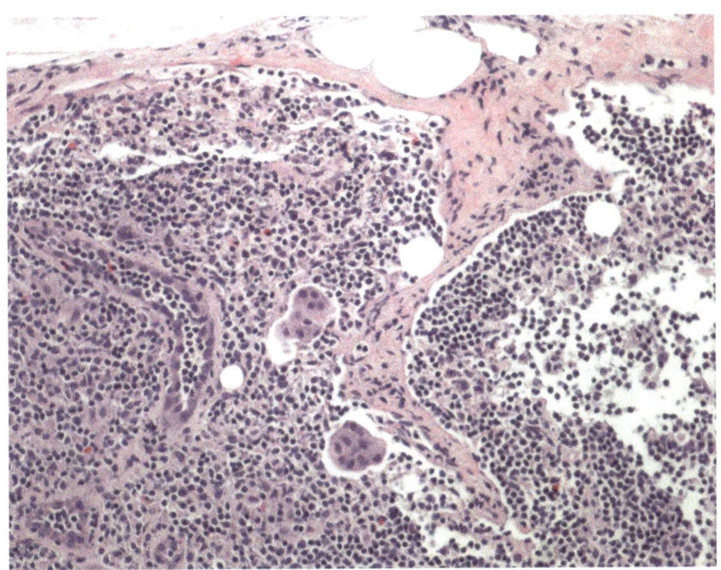

FIGURE 1.30 Low sensitivity of FS to detect small metastases. Permanent section of a SLN, which was negative on frozen section (see Fig. 1.29). Two small clusters of metastatic cells are present in the subcapsular sinus. This case illustrates the limitation of frozen section of SLN.

TABLE 1.2 A brief overview of the studies looking at the value of FS of SLN in lobular carcinomas.

Authors	Sample size	Sensitivity (%)	Accuracy (%)
Chan et al.	664	52	81
Horvath et al.	131	67	86
Leidenius et al.	100	72	87
Taras et al.	66	44	70
Turner et al.	27	18	66

methods for permanent section evaluation with variations in the number of H&E levels, serial versus step sectioning with defined intervals of 25–100 microns, single versus multiple levels used for keratin immunostaining, use of different types of keratin antibodies, etc. The permutations of these variations make it very difficult to reliably compare different studies. Although several meta-analyses have been published on this topic, the readers are cautioned in interpreting such studies.

TABLE 1.3 List of relatively larger studies assessing the value of FS in SLN in breast cancer.

Authors	Sample size	Sensitivity (%)	Specificity (%)	Accuracy (%)
Schrenk et al.	2326	65	100	88
McLaughlin et al.	931	56	100	85
Weiser et al.	890	58	99	89
Mitchell et al.	858	62	100	89
Langer et al.	648	64	100	87
Van de Vrande et al.	615	72	100	91
Wada et al.	569	84	100	95
Gemignani et al.	375	56	100	91
Leidenius et al.	375	83	99	93
Reitsamer et al.	328	81	100	93
Arora et al.	327	63	99	90
Liu et al.	326	68	100	90

A comprehensive list of all the studies that have looked at the value of FS in SLN is beyond the scope of this text, but a summary of some of the larger studies is provided in Table 1.3.

In summary, FS technique offers specificity approaching 100% though its sensitivity varies from 55 to 85% to detect metastases. It is reasonable to state that irrespective of the method adopted by an individual laboratory, the specificity of FS for SLN in breast is extremely high and reproducible.

Finally, FS tends to be more expensive as compared to TIC. In one of several studies on this topic, the difference in cost was nearly three times more for FS than TIC. In the current cost containment environment, this should be a consideration for every laboratory.

TOUCH IMPRINT CYTOLOGY (TIC) PREPARATION

The method to prepare TIC slides is relatively straight forward as compared to FS. It has minimal variables and time commitment. After the SLN has been adequately sliced, the cut surfaces are gently touched on a clean slide (touch imprint) or scraped off (smear preparation). The next step depends on the choice of staining method. Diff-quik is a rapid staining method for air-dried slides. In general, the cytoplasmic characteristics are better seen in such preparations. The other option is to fix the TIC slides in alcohol and use a rapid H&E stain. In addition, several other stains have also been utilized in different studies including Romanovsky, Giemsa, Papanicolaou, Toluidine blue, etc. The choice of these

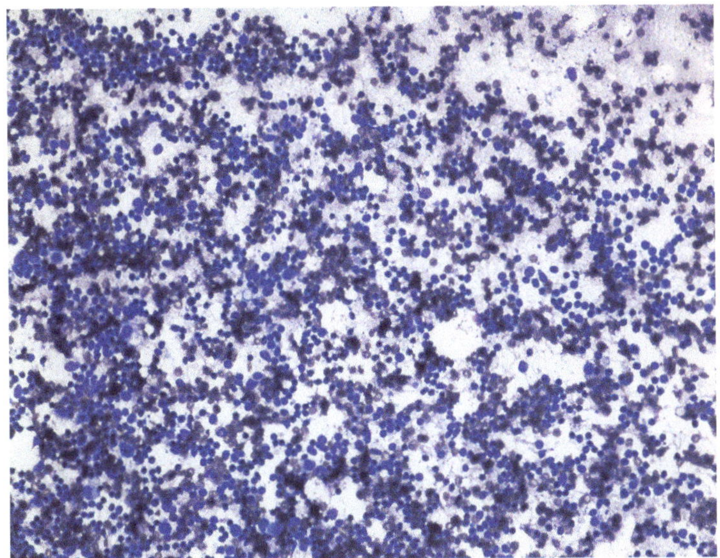

FIGURE 1.31 Touch imprint from a negative SLN. The imprint from SLN was air-dried and stained with diff-quik. There is a uniform sheet of small lymphocytes and red blood cells. No epithelial cells are identified.

staining methods rests with the individual laboratory and often remains discretion of the pathologist.

TIC EVALUATION OF SLN

The evaluation of TIC slides should follow a methodical and careful approach. The initial screening should be done on a scanning objective to get a general idea about overall cellularity of the preparation. At this power, one should look for clusters of cells. If present, then a high power evaluation can focus on these clusters of cells. The lymphocytes in the background serve as a control for tumor cell size (Figs. 1.31–1.40). The lymphocytes from the follicles often imprint as three-dimensional clusters but they lack any significant amount of cytoplasm and show individual large cells, as compared to clusters in case of metastatic carcinoma. Both diff-quik and rapid H&E stains clearly show the cytoplasm of epithelial cells. If clusters are not seen, then the slide should be carefully evaluated for single malignant epithelial cells. Again, the knowledge about the histologic type of the invasive tumor is very helpful in evaluating TIC of SLN (Table 1.4).

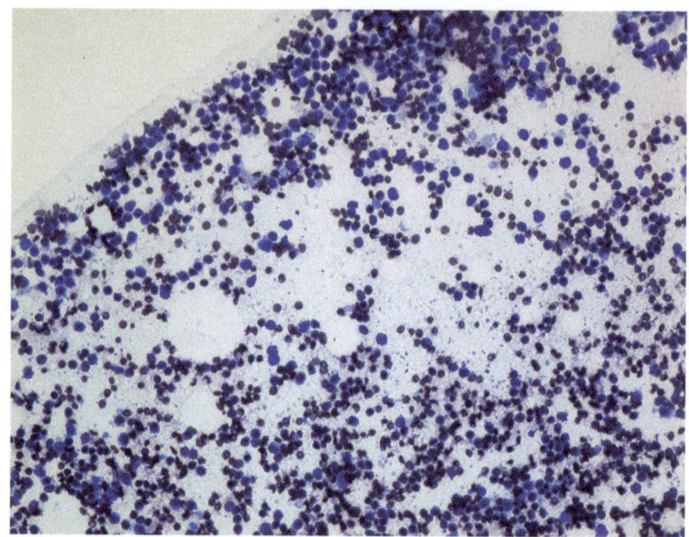

FIGURE 1.32 Touch imprint of a negative SLN. This is another example of diff-quik stained imprint of SLN, which does not show any metastatic tumor cells.

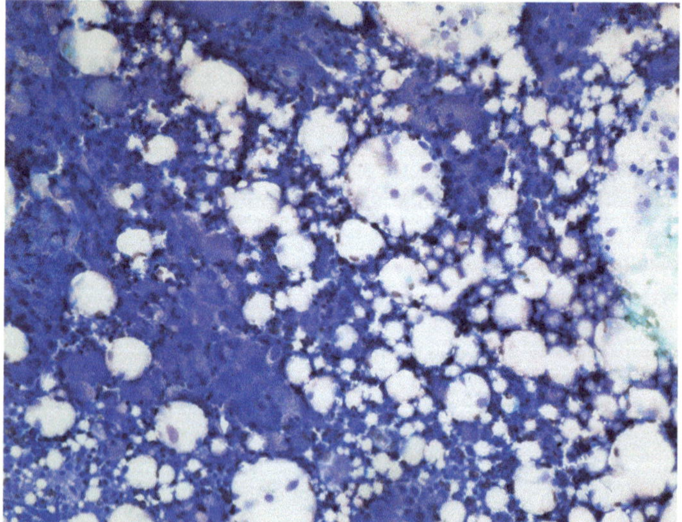

FIGURE 1.33 Air-dried touch imprint from a positive SLN. This imprint is slightly over air-dried and thick. Even then, it is easy to identify clusters of large epithelial cells, consistent with metastatic involvement.

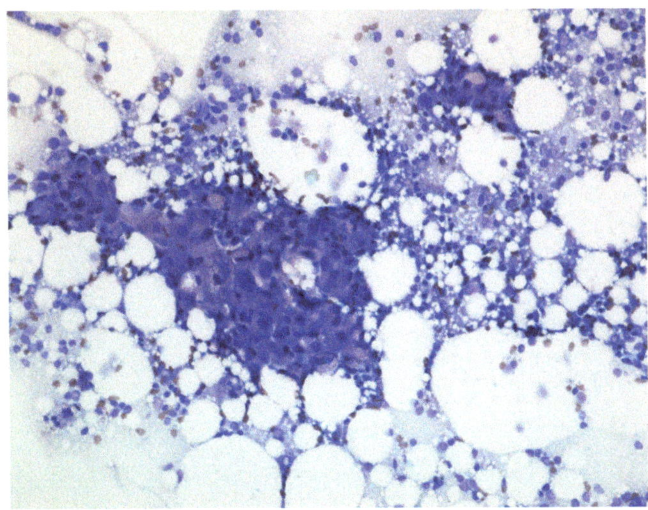

FIGURE 1.34 Diff-quik stained touch imprint from a positive SLN. This air-dried preparation is well prepared. The background shows some red cells. It is easy to identify a cluster of malignant epithelial cells.

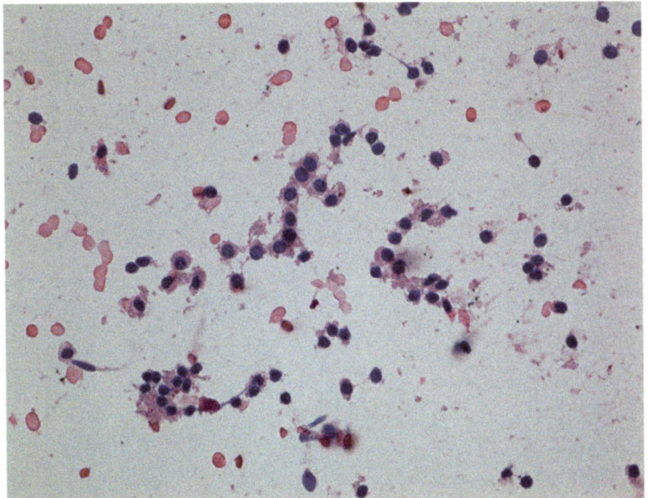

FIGURE 1.35 Touch imprint of a negative SLN. This is an alcohol fixed touch imprint of the SLN, stained with H&E. The background is relatively clear with a few red blood cells. The lymphocytes are easy to recognize. No epithelial cells are seen.

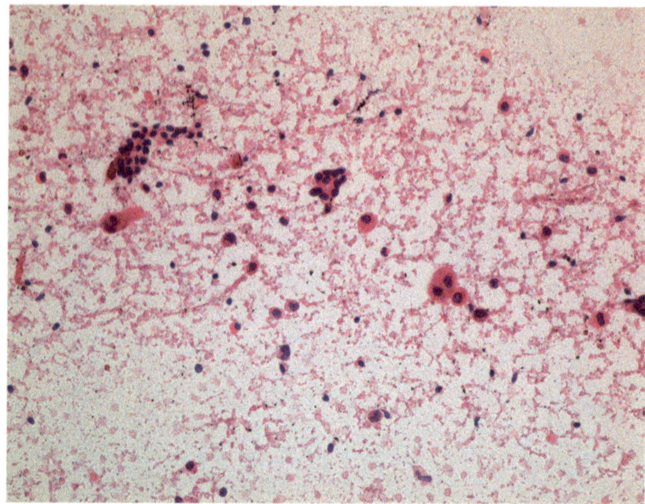

FIGURE 1.36 Alcohol fixed touch imprint of a positive SLN. In this preparation, there is an equal proportion of single and clusters of malignant epithelial cells. These preparations provide more detailed nuclear features and the cytoplasm also tends to stand out more as compared to air-dried preparations.

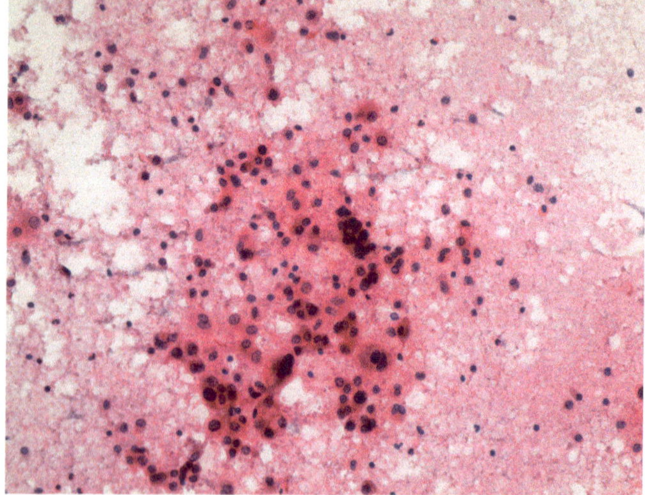

FIGURE 1.37 H&E stained touch imprint of a positive SLN. The background shows a few lymphocytes. The metastatic cells are loosely cohesive and have eosinophilic cytoplasm. Some single epithelial cells are also present.

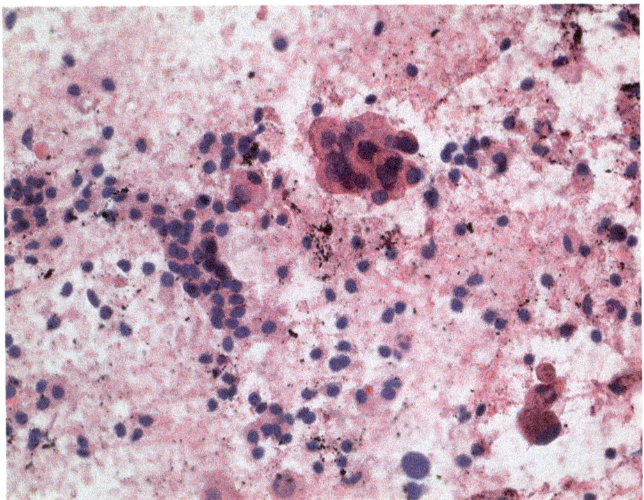

FIGURE 1.38 High power view of touch imprint of a positive SLN. In the background of predominantly small lymphocytes, the epithelial cells stand out as clusters of cells with dense cytoplasm. It is still easy to identify metastatic cells from a low nuclear grade tumor.

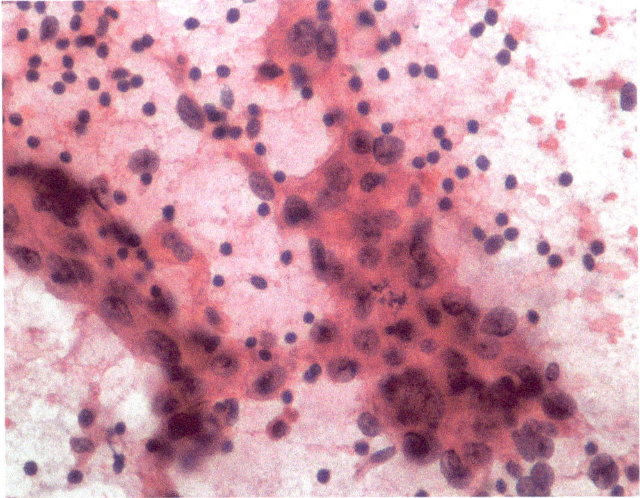

FIGURE 1.39 Touch imprint of a SLN with metastatic high-grade carcinoma. Metastases from a grade 3 ductal carcinoma are easy to find in imprint slides. Notice the marked nuclear pleomorphism and a mitotic figure.

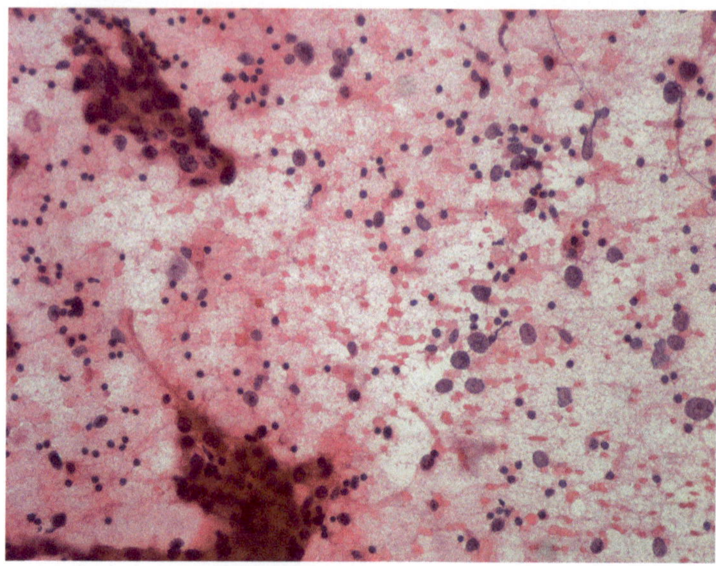

FIGURE 1.40 High power view of touch imprint of a positive SLN. This alcohol fixed touch imprint shows single as well as clusters of a high-grade metastatic ductal carcinoma. The tumor cells are 3–6 times larger than the lymphocytes.

TABLE 1.4 Key cytologic features in assessing touch imprint cytology of SLN.

- The information about the primary tumor, such as histologic type and grade should be available to the pathologist prior to evaluating the SLN
- Scan the section at low power to assess overall quality and cellularity of the preparation
- First look for clusters of cells and then perform a closer examination of such groups
- Besides the metastatic cells, lymphocytes can also appear in three-dimensional groups
- On diff-quik stained slides, the epithelial cells, both single cells and clusters stand out due to prominent cytoplasm, unlike lymphocytes.
- Cytoplasmic features, such as vacuoles or microacini of epithelial cells are easier to identify on air dried slides
- On H&E and other alcohol fixed slides, the epithelial cells often show dense pink cytoplasm and nuclear details are better appreciated

TABLE 1.5 Studies evaluating the utility of touch imprint cytology in assessing SLN in breast cancer.

Authors	Sample size	Sensitivity (%)	Specificity (%)	Accuracy (%)
Cox et al.	2137	53	99	85
Contractor et al.	896	73	100	93
Creager et al.	646	53	98	84
Teng et al.	507	62	100	87
Leidenius et al.	375	68	99	NA
Turner et al.	278	48	100	93
Henry-Tillman et al.	255	94	99	NA
Zgajnar et al.	250	34	99	72
Sauer et al.	211	51	98	NA
Barranger et al.	180	33	98	79

NA data not available

Besides the value of least amount of time to prepare TIC slides, a major advantage is no loss of tissue from SLN. This allows for more material to work with for permanent section histologic evaluation. As stated above, TIC is much cheaper to prepare as compared to FS. The potential disadvantages of TIC include relatively small number of cells available for evaluation, much larger time commitment and significant expertise on part of the pathologist interpreting these preparations and a higher chance of inability to make a definitive diagnosis.

Several studies have assessed the effectiveness of intraoperative TIC versus permanent section histology result and some studies have also compared TIC to FS in this setting. A summary of some of the larger studies on this topic is provided in Table 1.5.

These data suggest that the specificity of TIC is nearly as good as FS and often approaches 100%. The sensitivity is more variable from 33 to 94% as compared to FS. Finally, the accuracy of TIC is also lower in these studies than those reported with FS. It is important to keep in mind the differences in methodology in these studies and it is often difficult to make decisions at the individual laboratory level in selecting one or the other method. It is emphasized that the pathologists use their best clinical judgment in evaluating individual patients to provide the most reliable information to the surgeon.

MOLECULAR TECHNIQUES FOR INTRAOPERATIVE ASSESSMENT OF SLN

Unlike histologic and cytologic techniques, which have a significant element of sampling error, molecular techniques offer an ability to examine the entire specimen with potentially high sensitivity. However, traditionally these methods have suffered from low specificity. For intraoperative evaluation, two methods have been utilized, i.e., quantitative real-time polymerase chain reaction (qRT-PCR) and one-step nucleic acid amplification (OSNA).

The basic principles of molecular methods include homogenization of the entire tissue to be examined and reliance on detection of mRNA for gene products that are either uniquely expressed in the tumor cells or significantly overexpressed in the tumor cells as compared to the normal tissue. The disadvantage is lack of histological verification of the result. There have been some studies, where the tissue is equally divided into two halves; one half is used for a molecular assay and the other for histologic examination. However, this introduces sampling error, which often cannot be completely resolved.

For qRT-PCR technique, the focus has been on identifying a marker, which is only expressed in the tumor cells but not by non-neoplastic cells, and it is suitable to develop robust DNA probes. However, in breast cancer, such an ideal marker has not been identified. Therefore, two or more gene products are often utilized for these assays. Cytokeratin 19 and mammaglobin 1 have been the most frequently employed genes for this purpose. Despite the limitations, including high start up costs, time commitment and low specificity of qRT-PCR, several studies have assessed their utility in SLN (Table 1.6).

These studies confirm the higher sensitivity of qRT-PCR assays but demonstrate relatively lower specificity as compared to FS or

TABLE 1.6 Studies looking at sensitivity and specificity of qRT-PCR in SLN in breast cancer.

Authors	Sample size	Sensitivity (%)	Specificity (%)	Accuracy (%)
Blumencranz et al.	416	88	94	92
Veys et al.	367	89	95	94
Viale et al.	293	78	92	88
Cutress et al.	254	96	95	95

TABLE 1.7 List of a few studies that have evaluated the value of OSNA in SLN in breast cancer.

Authors	Sample size	Sensitivity (%)	Specificity (%)
Tamaki et al.	450	88	97
Visser et al.	346	95	95
Schem et al.	343	98	89

TABLE 1.8 Results from one of the studies comparing relative value of FS and TIC in breast cancer cases with or without neoadjuvant therapy (NAT).

	FS sensitivity	TIC sensitivity	FS specificity	TIC specificity	FS accuracy	TIC accuracy
No NAT	74	61	100	100	90	87
NAT	74	79	100	100	83	90

TIC. There is also an issue of false-positive results due to contamination. Unlike the research laboratories, frozen section suites are not often kept in a manner to substantially decrease contamination for such sensitive assays. So far, these assays have not been widely adopted in the clinical practice.

OSNA also detects mRNA but utilizes isothermal gene amplification. There is no denaturation step in OSNA and no meticulous extraction of RNA is required. OSNA employs six primers leading to increased specificity of this methodology over standard qRT-PCR. There is relatively limited data on the use of OSNA in SLN of breast and it is summarized in Table 1.7.

These early studies show promise of this technique, though more studies are needed to establish their value in the clinical practice.

SLN ASSESSMENT AFTER NEOADJUVANT THERAPY

In general, the identification of SLN after neoadjuvant therapy (NAT) is not problematic and the success rate for SLN mapping is similar to routine cases. The intraoperative assessment of SLN in this setting has been studied. Both the FS and TIC have been reported to be equally sensitive and specific and comparable to the data seen in cases without NAT. The results from a recent study comparing the two methods in these settings are summarized in Table 1.8.

FUTURE DIRECTIONS FOR INTRAOPERATIVE ASSESSMENT OF SLN

The premise of intraoperative evaluation of SLN has been to reduce the need for a second surgical procedure. Currently, the standard of practice has been to offer completion axillary lymph node dissection (ALND) in patients who are found to have positive SLN either during the primary surgical procedure or if the final pathology is positive for metastatic carcinoma. However, the recently reported results from American College of Surgeons Clinical Oncology Group (ACOSOG) Z0011 trial found that there was no statistically significant benefit from ALND for women who had clinically negative axilla but the SLN was positive. This is the first randomized clinical trial, which shows that patients with limited nodal metastasis in SLN do not gain any statistically significant survival advantage by adding ALND. Similar data has been seen in other studies, which show that in patients with limited or small metastasis in SLN, the removal and finding of a few additional positive axillary nodes often does not affect the decision for adjuvant therapy. Therefore, the role of intraoperative assessment of SLN in breast cancer seems to be in evolution. Either adoption of the findings of this study or other validation studies is likely to change the practice in this field.

Chapter 2
Assessment of the Surgical Margins

The local treatment of breast cancer has evolved significantly in the last 100 years. This was based on the notion that the removal of the entire breast and its lymphatic drainage area (axilla) would achieve not only local but also distant disease control. This Halstedian approach changed to modified radical mastectomy (MRM), when a better understanding developed that the treatment failure despite such a radical procedure was due to early dissemination of tumor cells, prior to surgical intervention. The pivotal study National Surgical Breast and Bowel Project (NSABP) B-04 showed equivalency of simple mastectomy plus radiation to MRM. A series of subsequent studies established that conservative surgery with whole breast radiation did not affect survival, as compared to total mastectomy (Table 2.1).

The National Institutes of Health (NIH) recommended breast conserving surgery (BCS) as the preferred surgical treatment for early breast cancer in 1991. Similarly, National Accreditation Center for Breast Cancer requires a BCS rate of at least 50%. The BCS rates have been reported to be as high as 90% in the published studies, but in general, most institutions reached the rates of about 65–70%. Recently, there has been an increase in mastectomy rates, which appears to be related to several factors, including genetic testing, improved breast reconstruction techniques, patient demand, and increased detection of multifocal tumor due to use of sensitive imaging modalities, such as magnetic resonance imaging (MRI).

The value of adequate surgical margin in decreasing local recurrence rates has been established both in invasive and in situ breast cancers. A summary of long-term studies looking at recurrence rates by margin status is provided in Table 2.2.

S.K. Mohsin, *Frozen Section Library: Breast*, Frozen Section Library 9,
DOI 10.1007/978-1-4614-0718-8_2,

TABLE 2.1 A summary of large prospective trials comparing survival after conservative breast surgery and radiation versus mastectomy.

Trial	Follow up (years)	Overall survival (%)	
		BCS + RT	Mastectomy
Milan	20	42	41
NSABP B-06	20	46	47
NCI	18	59	58
Institut Gustave-Roussy	15	73	65
EORTC	10	65	66

BCS + RT *breast conserving surgery + radiation therapy,* NSABP *National Surgical Adjuvant Breast and Bowel Project,* NCI *National Cancer Institute,* EORTC *European Organization for Research and Treatment of Cancer*

TABLE 2.2 Local recurrence rates by margin status in breast cancer.

Study site	No. of patients	Follow-up (year)	Recurrence rates by margin status (%)		
			Negative	Close	Positive
Fox Chase	1,262	6.3	7	14	12
Netherlands	1,026	6.5	2	6	16
Univ. of Penn	1,021	6.1	8	17	10
Yale	984	13	2	2	18
Gustave-Roussy	757	9	6	NA	14
Tufts	498	10	5	9	17
Stanford	289	6	2	16	9
Duke	259	3.8	2	NA	10

NA data not available

The local management of breast cancer continues to change and at the present time, BCS is the most common approach in all early breast cancers, typically detected by screening mammography. The goal of the breast surgeon is to get clear margins in one surgical procedure, whenever possible. A second surgical procedure is not desirable due to patient discomfort, costs, and risks associated with anesthesia and major surgery. Therefore, the evaluation of surgical margins during the surgical procedure is desirable by the surgeon. However, dealing with fatty breast tissue is difficult for the pathologist. Over the years, the pathologists have tried at least three methods for intraoperative margin assessment: gross examination after slicing the specimen, frozen section (FS), and touch imprints (TI). There has been variable success using these methods and the field of intraoperative assessment of surgical margins of breast specimens has evolved. In general, the surgeons have changed their practice from completely relying on intraoperative pathologic assessment to better preoperative and intraoperative imaging modalities to obtain adequate surgical margins.

GROSS EXAMINATION FOR SURGICAL MARGINS

In cases with a palpable mass, a careful gross examination after the specimen has been inked and thinly sliced, should allow the pathologist to assess the margins. A combination of close inspection and gentle palpation helps demarcate the extent of the tumor (Fig. 2.1). The margins can then be measured and reported to the surgeon. This method has not been reliable in accurately identifying the distance of the tumor to surgical margins. In one of the studies of 181 patients, followed for 5 years, grossly positive margins were associated with 21% local recurrence rate, as compared to cases with negative margins showing no recurrence. In another study of 254 patients, spread over a 6-year period, tumor within

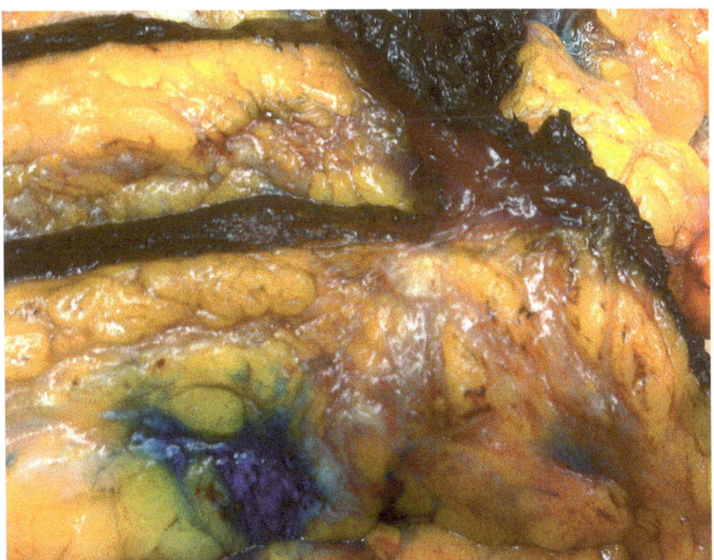

FIGURE 2.1 Invasive tumor involving the deep margin and pectoralis muscle. There is an irregular tumor mass in this mastectomy specimen. The *blue dye* represents injection at the previous lumpectomy site, used for sentinel node mapping. The tumor is very close to black-inked deep margin. A small piece of *brown* pectoralis muscle is present, as tumor abuts the fascia at this focus.

2 mm of the inked surface was considered margin-positive and >2 mm as margin-negative. Gross examination in this series did not accurately reflect the final margin status in 25% of the cases, when compared to the margin status in the final pathology report. Therefore, the surgical margin evaluation by gross examination alone has limited value in intraoperative assessment. However, in selected cases with well-demarcated, single tumor focus, 3–5-mm rim of normal appearing adipose tissue can be reliably considered as a negative margin. In most cases, the information that tumor is very close to the margin, may be sufficient for the surgeon to obtain additional tissue during the first surgical procedure. However, certain locations, such as anterior margin in a centrally located tumor, tumors close to medial edge of breast and in some cases tumor close to the inframammary crease may not leave much tissue to remove with good cosmesis. In such cases, an accurate assessment of close margins can be of significant value to the surgeon and the patient and other methods to evaluate the surgical margins, e.g., FS or TI should be considered.

FROZEN SECTION FOR SURGICAL MARGINS

It is difficult to obtain good sections of fat around the tumor and complete reliance on FS alone can lead to an erroneous interpretation of margin, i.e., closer than the actual distance. Tumors within 2–3 mm of the inked margins can be evaluated by frozen section. When mainly fibrous tissue is present around the tumor, then the likelihood of an accurate assessment of distance between the tumor and the margin is high (Figs. 2.2–2.8). On the other hand, normal adipose tissue around the tumor would most likely result in an underestimation of true distance to the margin (Figs. 2.9–2.11). In both these cases, a relatively small piece of tissue with tumor should be placed in a larger sized tissue disc to allow for a rim of OCT gel, which can be very helpful in obtaining a good section. Another helpful point is to consider cutting the FS at a thickness of 8–9 mm, in order to get reasonable complete sections (Fig. 2.12). During the process of FS, evaluation of frozen tissue in the cryostat, after the frozen tissue block has been faced can be very helpful to see the relationship between the tumor, which appears white or gray-white against bright yellow adipose tissue and the inked surface (Figs. 2.13 and 2.14). The advantage of a good frozen section is that it allows measurements of margins in millimeters rather than a qualitative assessment as positive or negative. The reliability of FS in assessing surgical margins in breast cancer has been reported in a few studies (Table 2.3). This limited data suggest that FS can be a fairly reliable method for surgical margin assessment.

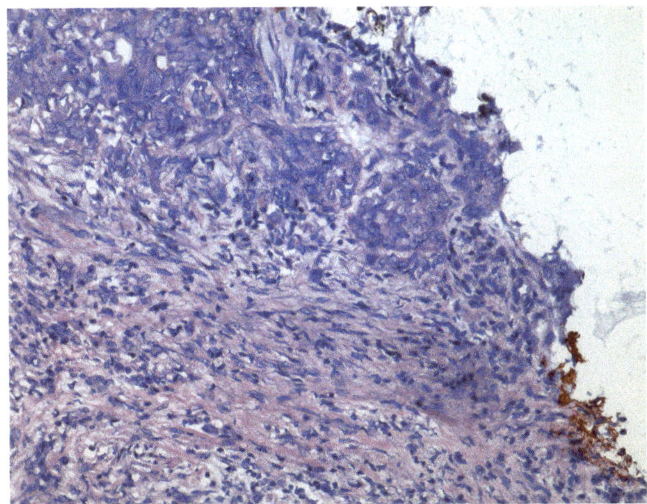

FIGURE 2.2 An invasive tumor is transected at the margin. There is significant frozen artifact in the tumor cells but they are recognizable, as compared to inflammatory cells elsewhere in the section.

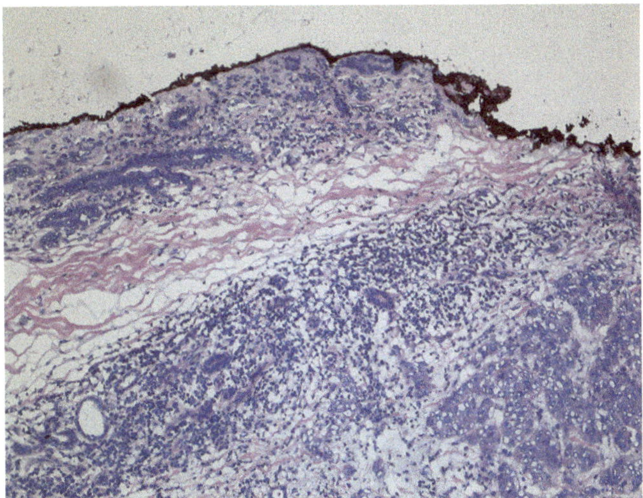

FIGURE 2.3 Very close margin on frozen section. This is a high power view of section from Fig. 2.2. There is an inflamed normal breast unit at the inked margin.

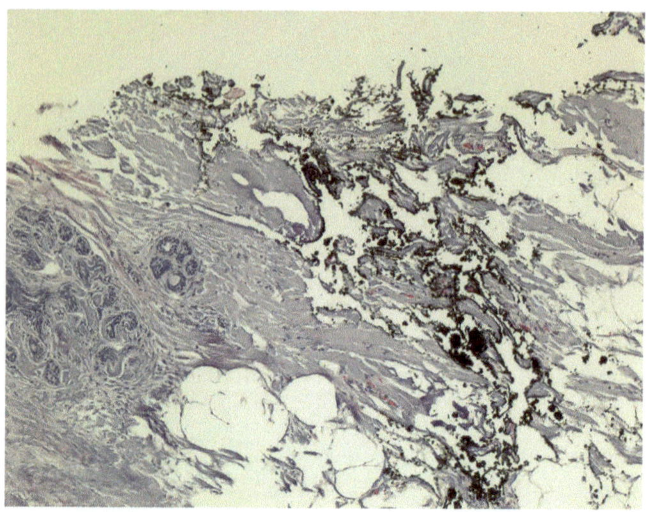

FIGURE 2.4 Negative margin on frozen section. The tissue is fragmented and ink has seeped into the tissue. However, the histologic features are easy to read and show benign breast epithelium and stroma.

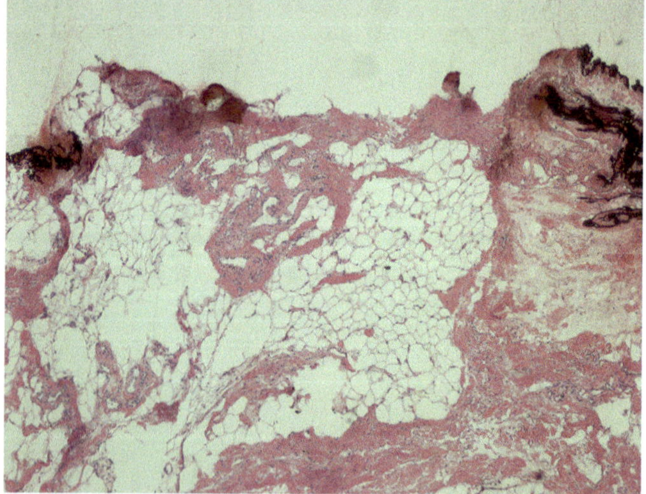

FIGURE 2.5 Optimal frozen section due to fibrous tissue at the margin. Due to less fat in the tissue, an optimal section can be prepared and it shows negative surgical margin.

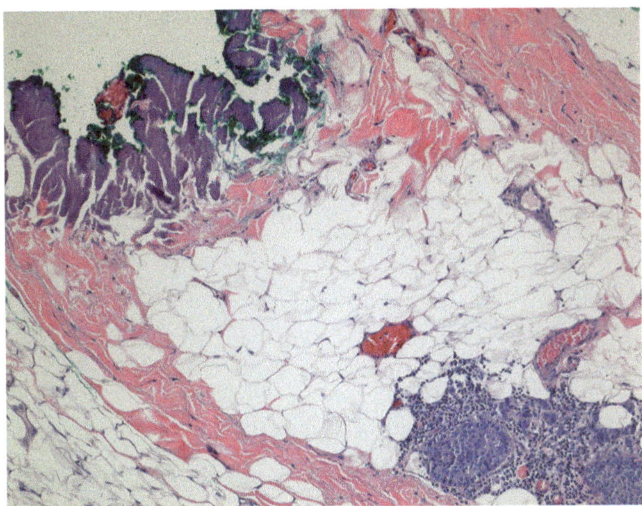

FIGURE 2.6 Close but negative margin on frozen section. The inked and cauterized margin is present in the left upper corner. There is a small focus of DCIS and associated invasive tumor with fat between the tumor and the inked margin. Therefore, the margin is negative but close.

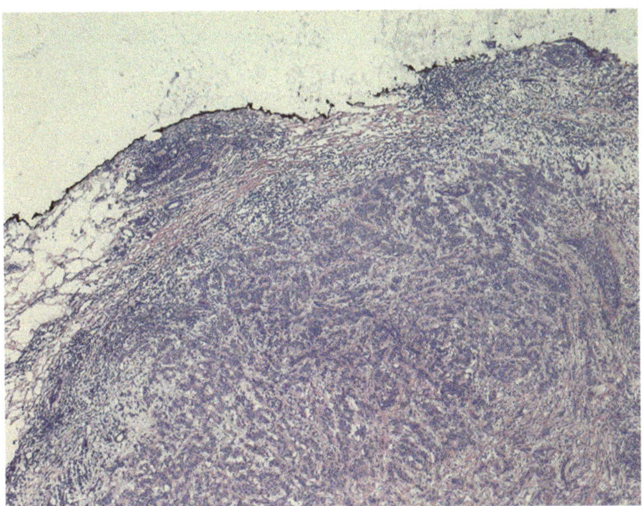

FIGURE 2.7 Close margin for invasive tumor on frozen section. The invasive tumor has a relatively circumscribed edge and it is within 1 mm of the inked margin. It appears that there is rim of benign tissue at the margin.

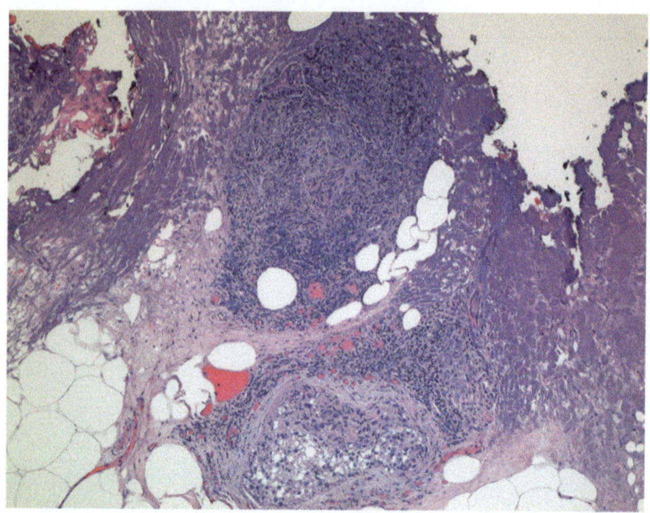

FIGURE 2.8 Indeterminate margin on frozen section. There is marked cautery artifact with crushed cells, which cannot be reliably interpreted. There is a small intact focus of DCIS. On close examination, it appears that DCIS is very close to the margin and there is a piece of cauterized epithelium on the left. Overall, the margin evaluation is indeterminate in this case.

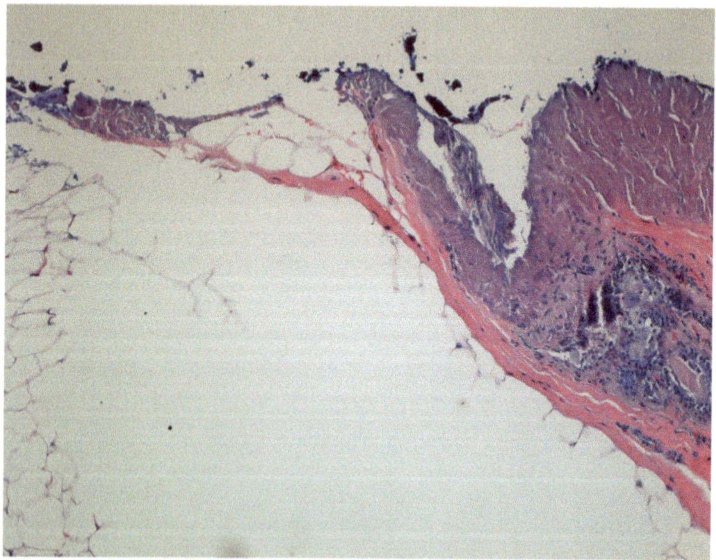

FIGURE 2.9 The main limitation of frozen section for margins is inability to obtain complete sections of fatty tissue. This is a fairly good quality frozen section showing small amount of benign breast epithelium in fibrous stroma. However, most of the fatty tissue is missing in the section.

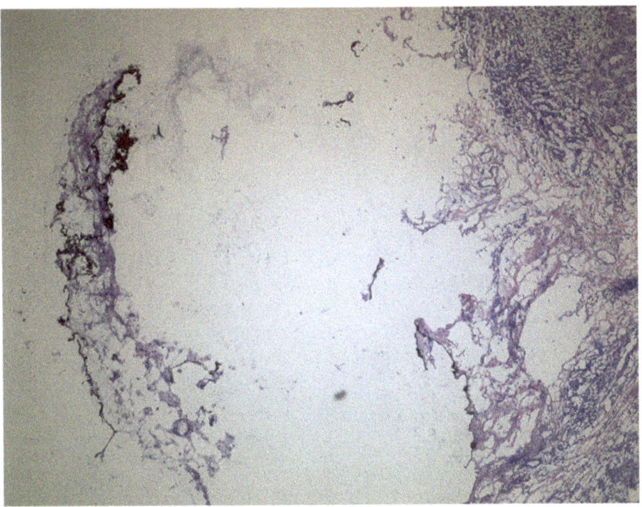

FIGURE 2.10 Difficult frozen section due to fat. Due to mainly fat, there is a large piece of tissue missing in this section. The tumor is on the right and there is some benign breast tissue after the tumor. The margin can be reported as negative with confidence; however, the actual distance cannot be measured in frozen section.

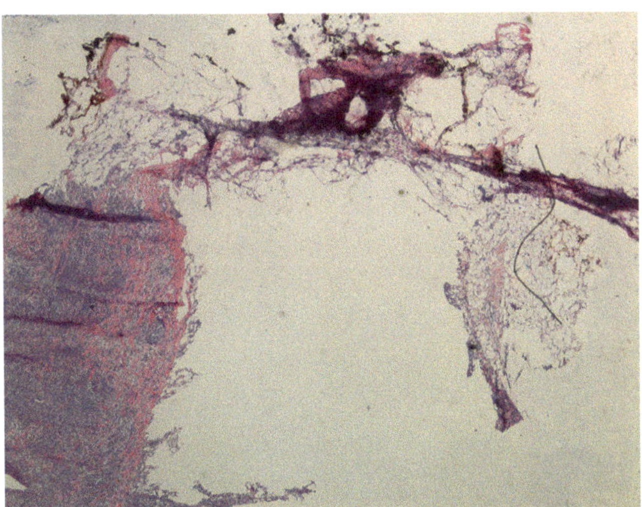

FIGURE 2.11 Fatty tissue at the margin precludes reliable assessment of the actual surgical margin. The tissue has folded over due to pure fat between the tumor and the inked surface. The margin appears negative but it is impossible to measure the exact distance between the tumor and the actual margin.

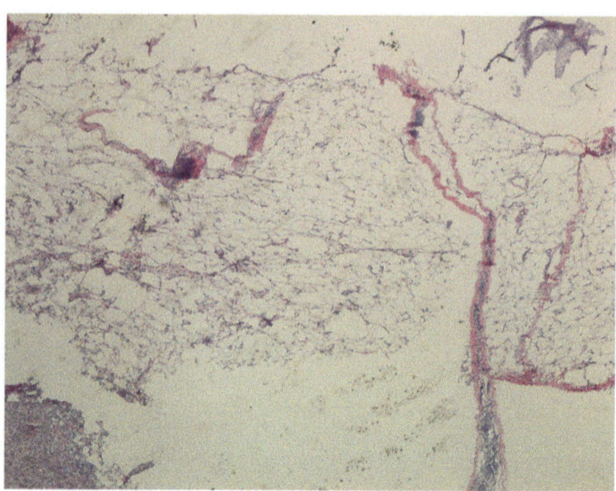

FIGURE 2.12 Technique to cut full sections of fatty tissue. One of the ways to obtain reasonable quality section of fatty breast tissue is to increase the section thickness in the cryostat. In the section illustrated here, the section was cut at 8-mm thickness, leading to a fairly complete section of fat. The tumor is seen at the bottom and true distance between the tumor and the inked margin can be measured.

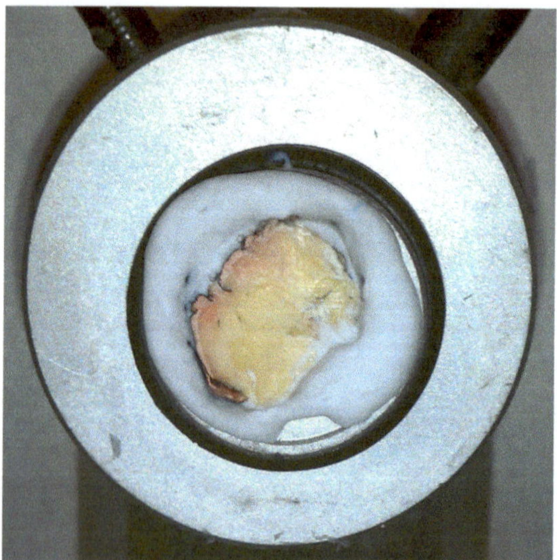

FIGURE 2.13 Examination of the frozen tissue block in cryostat. This is a trimmed frozen section block for margin evaluation. The examination of block in the cryostat is a helpful adjunct during the intraoperative assessment. One can see that the entire tissue is composed of fat and the possibility of getting a good frozen section is very low.

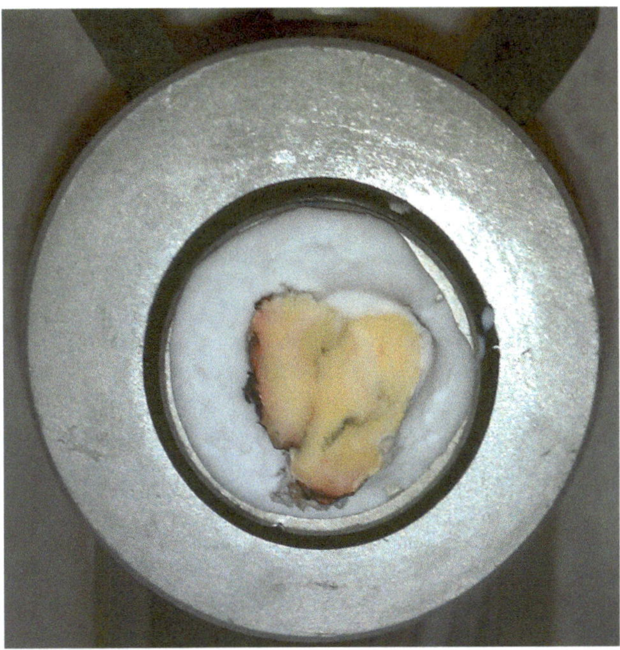

FIGURE 2.14 Examination of the frozen tissue block in cryostat. A close examination of trimmed frozen tissue block is very helpful in studying the topography of margin and rest of the tissue. In this case, the tissue appears to be fibrous at the margin. The frozen section preparation is expected to be reasonable.

TABLE 2.3 Studies evaluating the utility of frozen section in assessing surgical margins in breast cancer.

Authors	No. of patients	Sensitivity (%)	Specificity (%)
Olson et al.	290	90	100
Weber et al.	140	91	100

TOUCH IMPRINT FOR SURGICAL MARGINS

Touch imprint or preparation of the surgical margin is another way to perform intraoperative margin assessment. An appropriately labeled glass slide is touched to each of the five or six surfaces, depending on whether there is any attached skin to obtain cells for evaluation. A simple and quick stain, such as Diff-quik or Toluidine blue can be used on air-dried slides. For surfaces, measuring more than 5 cm, two imprints are prepared for each surface to adequately sample the surgical margin. The other options include use of rapid H&E or Papanicolaou stain on alcohol-fixed slides. The slides are then screened to look for malignant epithelial cells. This method yields either no epithelial cells or rare clusters of benign epithelial and nonepithelial cells, when the margin is negative versus atypical or malignant epithelial cells in case of a positive margin (Figs. 2.15–2.25). This method has been successfully used by several laboratories, and on average takes about 10 min per specimen. Some of the studies that have evaluated the value of TI in evaluating surgical margins are summarized in Table 2.4. These studies suggest that the use of TI in this setting is not highly reproducible and has low sensitivity in low-grade tumors. This may be related to differences in technique and lack of expertise among interpreting pathologists. However, Moffitt Cancer center in a series of publications has shown this to be reproducible in their hands and their long-term follow-up study on 701 patients showed a low recurrence rate of 2.7% at 3.5 years

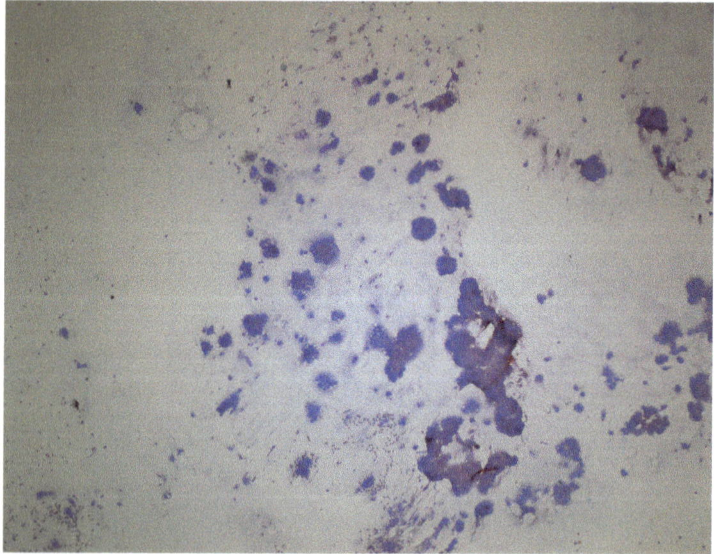

FIGURE 2.15 Low power screening of imprint cytology preparation for margin evaluation. This is an air-dried preparation for margin evaluation, stained with diff-quik. The low power examination at scanning objective is extremely useful. This imprint slide is very cellular and shows cell clusters of variable size and shape, consistent with positive margin.

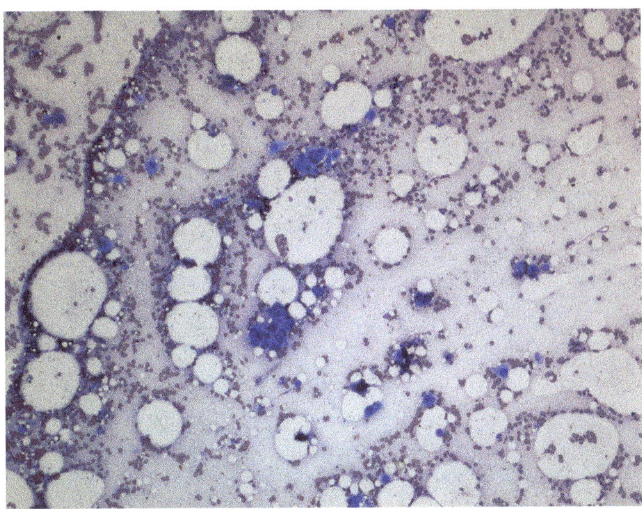

FIGURE 2.16 Rare tumor cells on touch imprint. This touch imprint shows blood in the background with relatively few single and small clusters of malignant epithelial cells. Careful screening of such preparations is needed in order to reach the correct diagnosis.

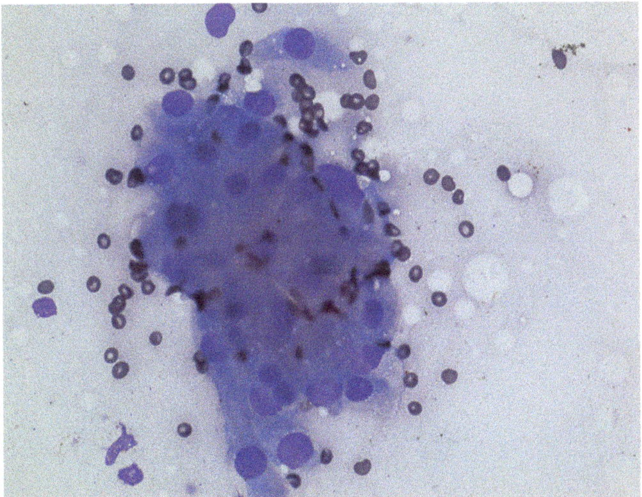

FIGURE 2.17 Positive imprint from surgical margin. This high power view shows a cluster of epithelial cells with malignant cytologic features, e.g., enlarged cells, nucleomegaly, high NC ratio and nucleolus. There is some cellular dyscohesion.

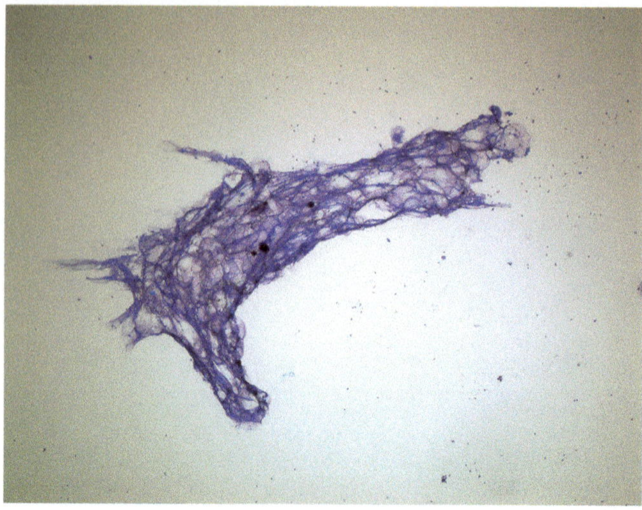

FIGURE 2.18 Negative margins on diff-quik stained imprint. This air-dried imprint from a surgical margin shows a piece of benign adipose tissue. No epithelial cells are present, consistent with negative margin.

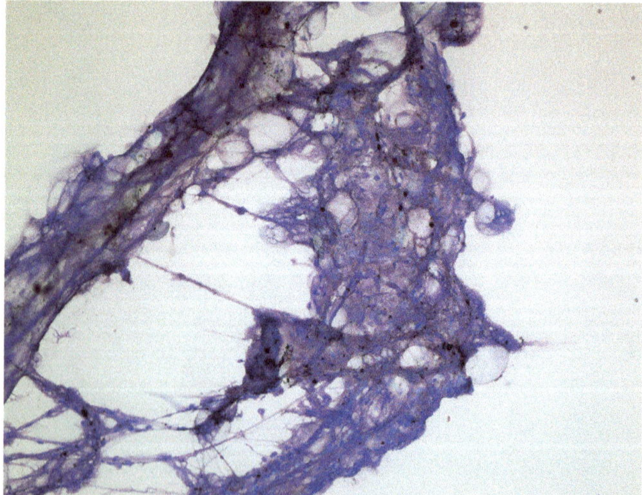

FIGURE 2.19 Typical appearance of imprint from a negative margin. There is a large piece of adipose tissue in a clean background. This is a fairly typical appearance of touch imprints in case of a negative margin.

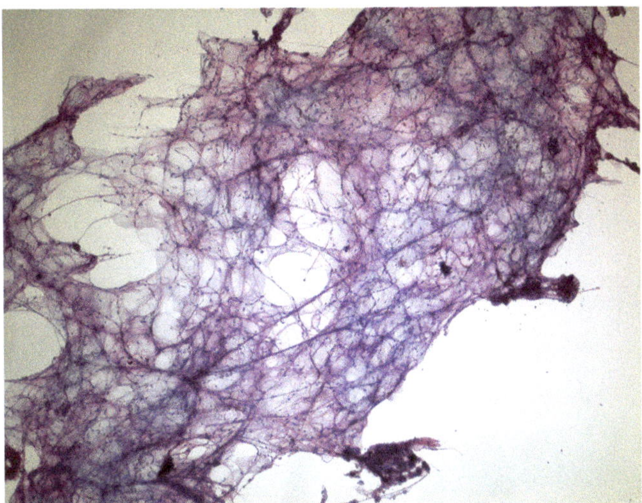

FIGURE 2.20 Touch imprint from normal breast tissue at margin. This slide shows a clean background with a large fragment of adipose tissue. There are a few possible clusters of epithelial cells, which need more evaluation.

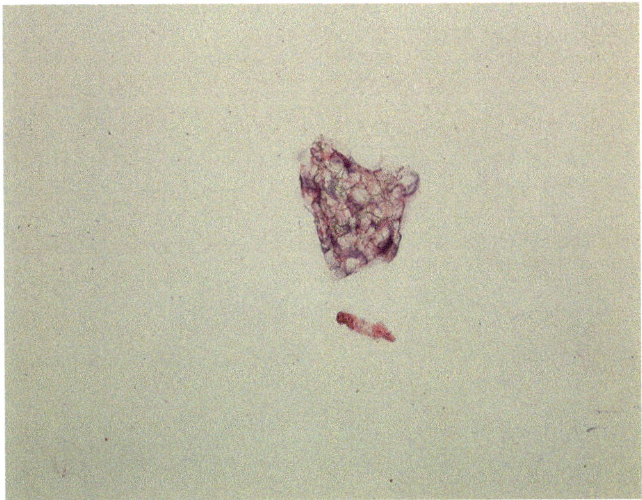

FIGURE 2.21 Alcohol-fixed touch imprint for surgical margin evaluation. This touch imprint for margin is fixed in alcohol and a rapid H&E stain is done. The background is clear and there is only a small amount of fat on the slide, consistent with a negative margin.

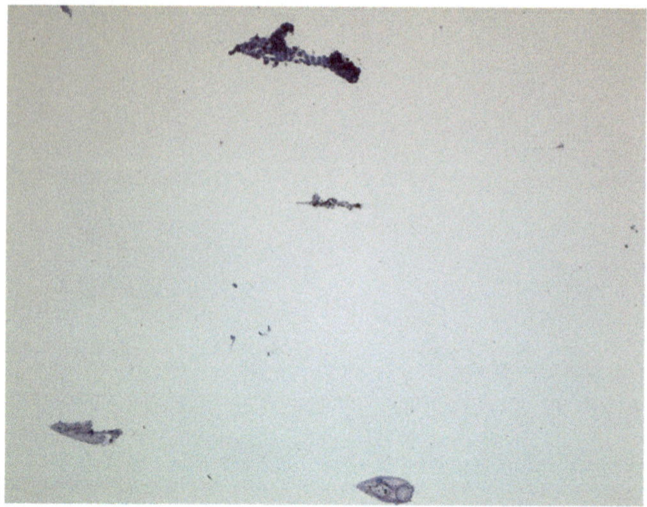

FIGURE 2.22 Typical features of touch imprint from a negative margin. Intermediate power view of an alcohol-fixed touch imprint. Besides clear background and small amount of fat, there is a small group of epithelial cells. They are arranged in monolayer and have uniform nuclei, typical of benign breast ductal epithelium. The interpretation is negative margin.

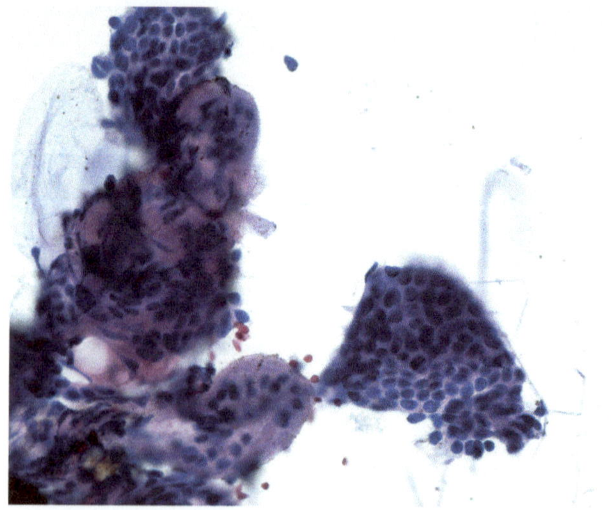

FIGURE 2.23 Evaluation of epithelial structures from touch imprints. High power view of the epithelial group seen in Fig. 2.24. Note the flat sheet-like arrangement, uniform nuclear size, and slightly branched architecture of normal ductal epithelium.

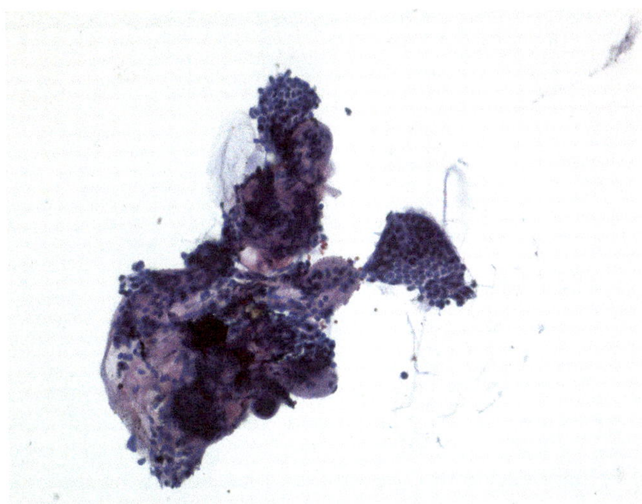

FIGURE 2.24 Evaluation of epithelial structures from touch imprints. Intermediate power view of normal breast epithelial component in a touch imprint. The overall architecture recapitulates a terminal duct lobular unit.

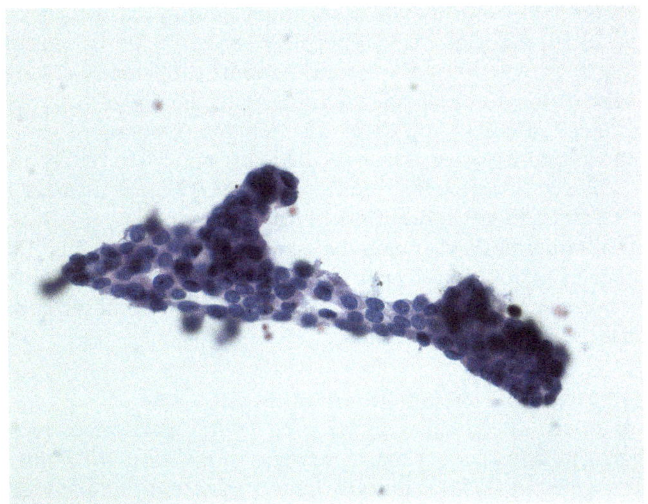

FIGURE 2.25 Normal breast epithelium on touch imprint of surgical margin. High power view of normal breast epithelial component (seen in Fig. 2.22), sometimes seen on touch imprints of negative margins.

TABLE 2.4 List of studies evaluating the usefulness of touch imprint method of surgical margin assessment.

Authors	No.	Sensitivity (%)	Specificity (%)
Klimberg et al.	428	100	100
D'Halluin et al.	400	89	92
Cox et al.	114	100	97
Saarela et al.	55	38	–
Valdes et al.[a]	12	8	98

[a] Invasive lobular carcinoma only

of median follow-up. Therefore, TI for margin assessment for breast specimens can be safe, rapid, and in experienced hands a relatively reliable method. Some reports state that touch imprint can be successful in the assessment of margin during second surgery to obtain clear margins. However, it is important to exercise caution in interpreting either TI or FS in this setting, since the changes after the initial surgery can mimic malignancy.

Some studies have specifically evaluated a combination of different methods in reducing the re-excision rates for positive margin at the time of the first surgery. Weber et al. compared the benefits of specimen radiography and FS in assessing surgical margins in 115 lesions. FS assessment of surgical margins rendered 27.5% cases as margin-negative versus 14.3% by specimen radiography only. In a series of 264 patients with stage 0–III breast cancers, Cabioglu et al. reported that with the use of intraoperative margin assessment, about 25% of this population was rendered margin-negative. They verified this approach by reporting the 5-year recurrence-free survival rate of 99% for invasive and 100% for DCIS after addition of radiation therapy to BCS. In another study of DCIS, using the same methodology, a significant number of patients were spared a second surgery to obtain negative margins. These studies demonstrate the benefit of intraoperative surgical margin assessment.

OTHER INDICATIONS FOR FROZEN SECTION

FS of breast specimens can be used in the assessment of skin margins in skin-sparing mastectomies. In addition, a FS may be used to rule out DCIS or invasive cancer in cases of nipple-sparing mastectomy. Usually a section from subareolar area is submitted for FS evaluation (Figs. 2.26–2.33). Unlike the FS for soft tissue margins for palpable or nonpalpable cancers, FS are technically

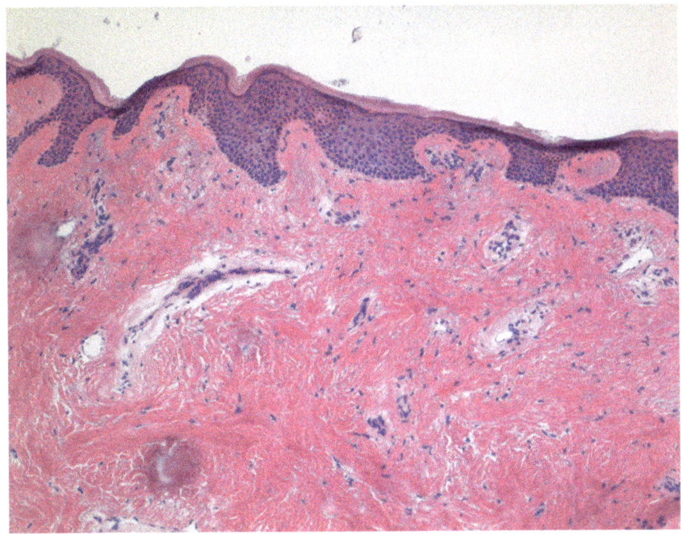

FIGURE 2.26 Frozen sections of skin margins in locally advanced cancer. They are easy to prepare and evaluate, unlike fatty breast tissue. Detailed histologic examination is possible. In this case, the margin is negative.

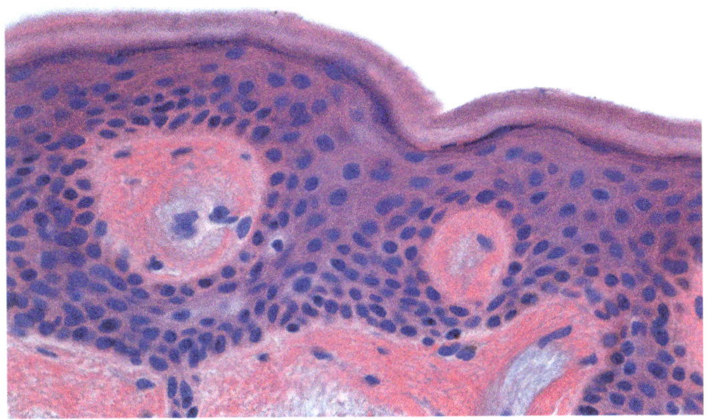

FIGURE 2.27 Skin margin for Paget's disease. Skin margin by frozen section. Another example of good microscopic details in the epidermis to rule out Paget's disease.

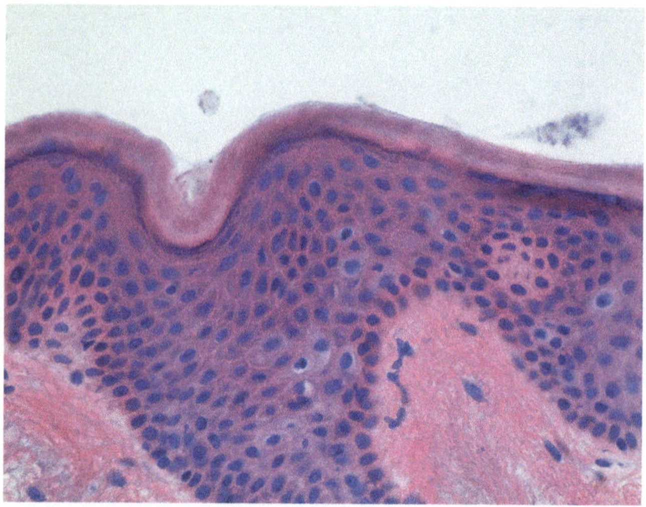

FIGURE 2.28 Skin margin for Paget's disease. High power view of skin margin for a case with Paget's disease. These sections are easy to cut and show enough details to easily rule out malignant cells in the epidermis.

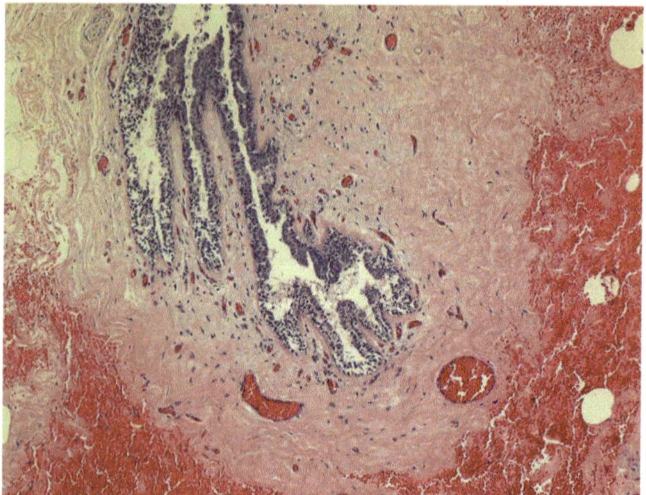

FIGURE 2.29 Frozen section of the subareolar area with a normal duct. There is some hemorrhage and the surgeon was concerned about biopsy site and thus tumor extending too close to nipple to prevent nipple-sparing mastectomy.

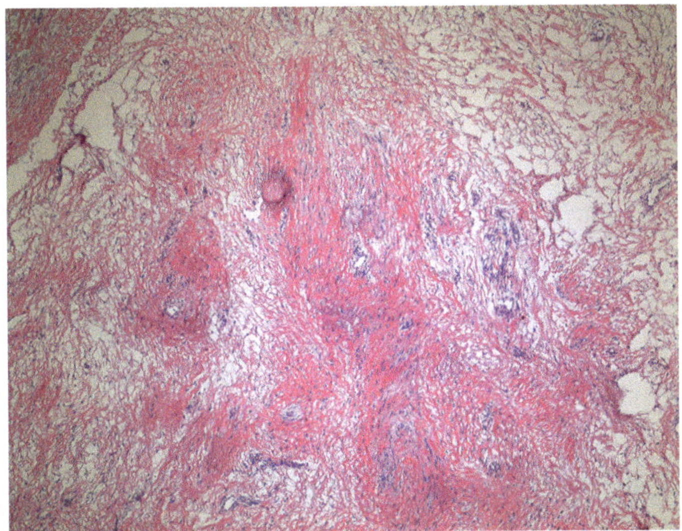

FIGURE 2.30 Frozen section to rule out DCIS extending into the nipple area. No large ducts are seen and the stroma appears benign.

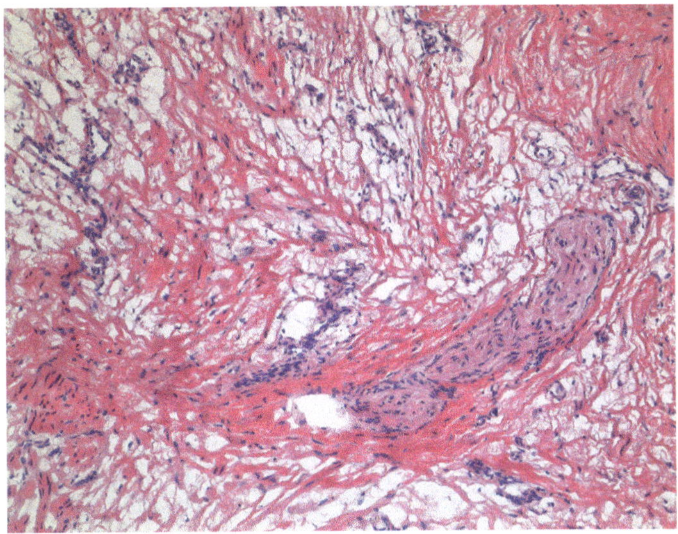

FIGURE 2.31 Frozen section of nipple area. A good quality frozen section allows for detailed examination of benign structures. A nerve and a few blood vessels are identified. No epithelial structures are seen.

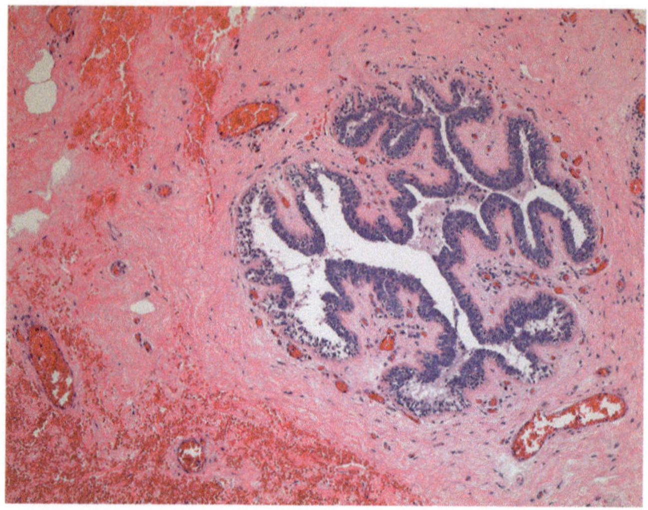

FIGURE 2.32 Frozen section of anterior margin for a centrally located tumor. A benign duct is seen in cross-section. No epithelial proliferation is noted.

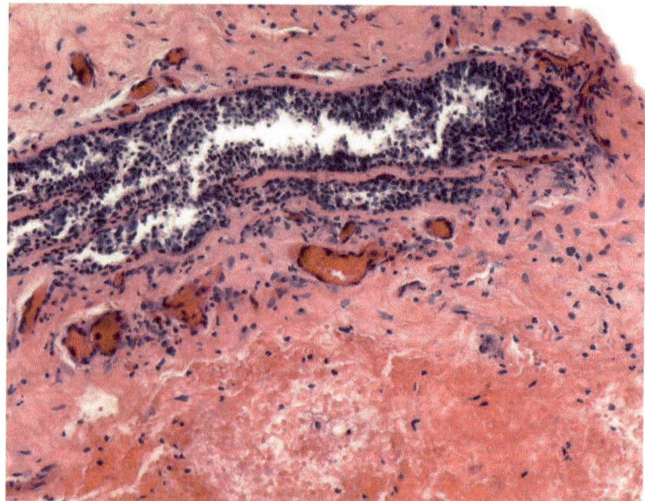

FIGURE 2.33 Frozen section of the subareolar tissue in nipple-sparing mastectomy. A segmental duct is cut longitudinally but shows the two layers without atypia.

easy to perform for evaluation of skin and nipple margins. In such cases, the FS evaluation is primarily used for the diagnosis of malignancy, i.e., DCIS or invasive cancer, particularly in nipple-sparing mastectomy. Certain benign lesions, such as radial sclerosing lesions, intraductal papillomas, sclerosing adenosis, and subareolar sclerosing duct hyperplasia can mimic either in situ or invasive carcinoma. Similarly, a small invasive lobular or tubular carcinoma in this location can be difficult to diagnose. FS artifacts can further enhance the difficulty in making a reliable diagnosis of benignity in these situations. In general, a conservative approach should be used.

Chapter 3
Diagnostic Evaluation of a Breast Mass

Increased awareness and education of the patients has led to improved detection of lumps or masses in the breast. They come to clinical attention in three common ways: (1) patient feels something during breast self-examination, (2) the primary care physician or gynecologist feels a lump during routine physical examination, or (3) screening mammography identifies a mass (Fig. 3.1). All these methods of finding a breast mass bring a lot of anxiety to the patient. A breast examination by a trained physician can often distinguish between benign versus worrisome lumps. Sometimes the changes associated with a breast mass, such as change in the size and appearance of the breast, skin dimpling, nipple retraction, nipple discharge, or skin color and tone, as compared to the other breast brings the problem to the attention of patient or their physician. A breast mass appears as density or distortion on the screening mammogram and the Breast Imaging-Reporting and Data System (BI-RADS) can classify the finding into benign, indeterminate, suspicious, or highly suspicious for malignancy.

In the majority of cases, additional workup, such as diagnostic mammogram and/or ultrasound leads to tissue sampling for diagnosis (Fig. 3.2). This can be either a fine needle aspiration (FNA) or minimally invasive percutaneous core biopsy. This leads to the definite diagnosis in most cases. The use of a specific type of diagnostic biopsy depends on patient, physician, and institutional preferences. FNA is relatively easy and quick to do and the diagnosis can be made rapidly; however, FNA may not distinguish between

S.K. Mohsin, *Frozen Section Library: Breast*, Frozen Section Library 9,
DOI 10.1007/978-1-4614-0718-8_3,

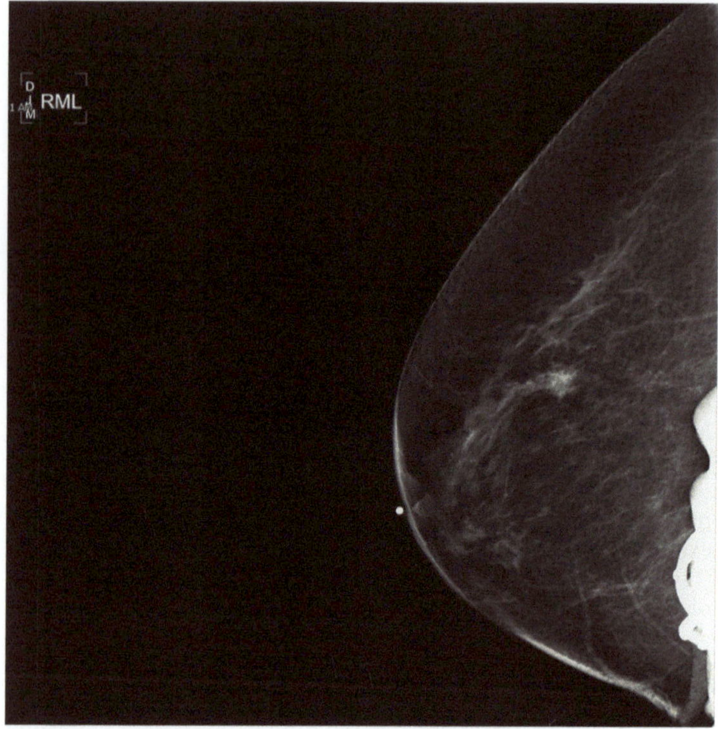

FIGURE 3.1 Diagnostic mammogram of an invasive tumor. This image from a postmenopausal women shows relatively radiolucent breast with a distinct, irregular, stellate lesion, characteristic of invasive cancer.

in situ versus invasive cancer. There are limitations on assessing biomarkers in such small samples as well. Some of the situations, where FNA can be very helpful are listed in Table 3.1. On the other hand, core needle biopsy provides histologic diagnosis and separation between in situ and invasive cancer. The testing of predictive biomarkers on core biopsies is fairly reliable and can be very useful in cases where neoadjuvant therapy is a consideration (Table 3.2).

Therefore, in the current practice, frozen section on lumpectomy or mastectomy is unusual. The most common indication is for the assessment of the surgical margins (this topic is covered in Chap. 2). The rest of the chapter focuses on handling of such specimens and gross assessment of a breast mass. After proper identification of the specimen, it should be weighed and measured in three dimensions. If there is any attached skin, then its appearance or any skin lesions should be described.

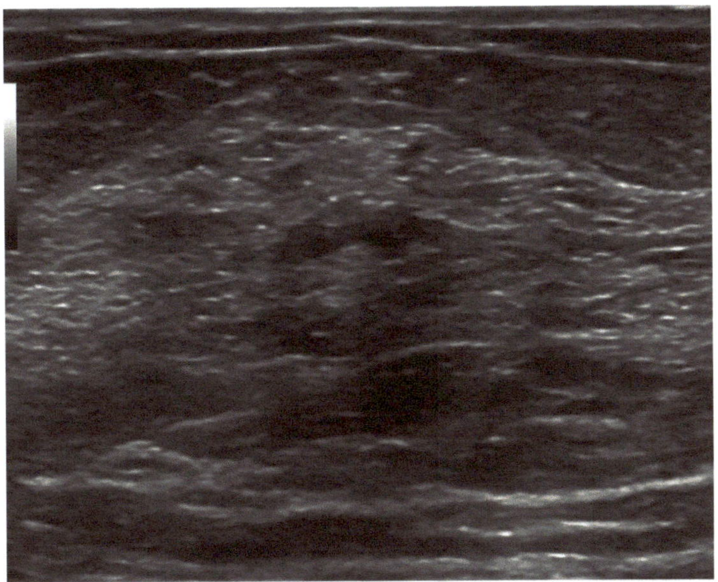

FIGURE 3.2 Ultrasound of a breast density seen on a diagnostic mammogram. There is an irregular, hypoechoic mass with irregular borders, wider than taller, and internal acoustic shadowing. These ultrasonographic features are diagnostic for an invasive carcinoma.

TABLE 3.1 Situations in which fine needle aspiration biopsy can be helpful.

- The palpable lump is clinically benign and FNA is to reassure the patient
- Patient is anxious and clinical breast examination is equivocal
- The lump is clinically very suspicious and patient prefers rapid diagnosis
- A positive FNA can be used to establish the diagnosis for precertification for an MRI; FNA introduces minimal artifact that can interfere with MRI reading
- A palpable and suspicious axillary lymph node can be sampled by FNA to confirm locally advanced breast cancer without requiring a surgical procedure

INKING OF BREAST SPECIMENS FOR SURGICAL MARGINS

The orientation of surgical specimen has been required as a quality measure by the American Society of Breast Surgeons (ASBS). Surgeons across the world have adopted a simple approach of

TABLE 3.2 Relative advantages of core needle biopsy in the diagnostic algorithm of a breast mass.

- It can be done right away at the time of diagnostic mammogram or ultrasound
- It provides relatively reliable information about the tumor, such as in situ or invasive cancer, histologic subtype, tumor grade, etc.
- It obtains sufficient tissue to assess biomarkers, if primary surgery is not possible
- Multifocal lesions can be sampled and diagnosed reliably, which can help with treatment planning
- Certain large gauge biopsy instruments can remove small benign lumps, thus potentially avoiding a surgical procedure

TABLE 3.3 Surgical margin identification inking scheme for breast lumpectomies.

Anterior	Orange
Posterior	Black
Superior	Purple
Inferior	Green
Medial	Blue
Lateral	Yellow

"short suture for superior" and "long suture for lateral" to orient the breast specimens. Based on the same principle, it is ideal to use a standardized method in the gross room for inking breast specimens. Currently, six pigment-based tissue-inking systems are available, in addition to India ink. Schemes for using these inks for breast specimens are provided in Table 3.3 and Figs. 3.3 and 3.4. The specimens should be inked fresh. It should be dried prior to applying inks. In general, cotton tipped applicators or small sponge brushes are preferred over paint brush, to avoid pushing the ink into fatty crevices on the specimen surface. After applying the inks, the surface should be sprayed with solution containing 5% acetic acid in water or a commercially available solution to make the inks stick to the tissue (Fig. 3.5). Any excess ink should be washed away prior to sectioning. Another option is the use of a sterile tissue inking kit by the surgeon immediately after removing the specimen from the breast, potentially decreasing the effects of any tissue distortion.

Lumpectomies and wire-guided excisions for nonpalpable lesions, performed in conjunction with sentinel lymph node

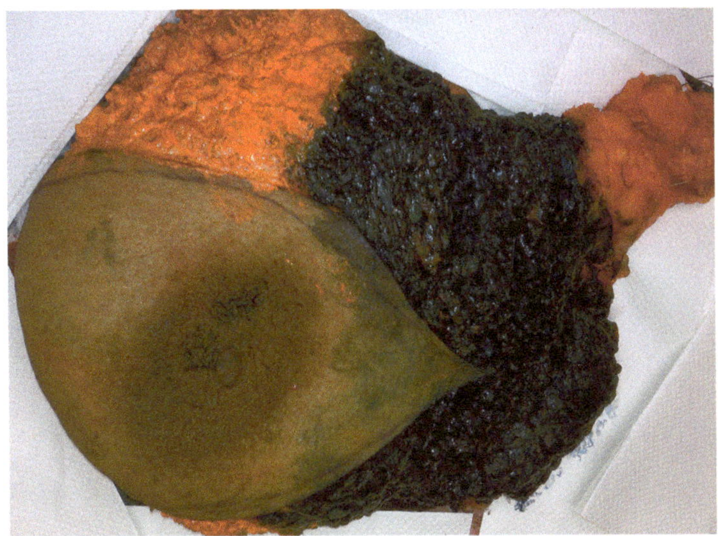

FIGURE 3.3 Surgical margin inking of a mastectomy specimen. The attached axillary contents in this modified radical mastectomy help orient the specimen. The lateral half is inked *blue* and the medial half with *orange* ink. No lesions are seen on the nipple, areola, or skin.

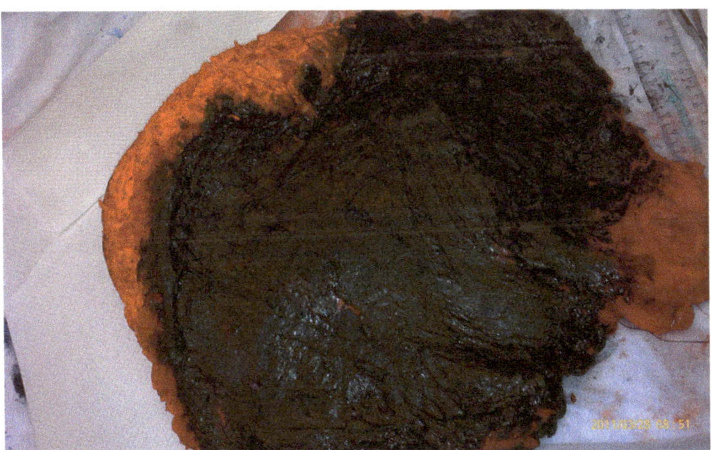

FIGURE 3.4 Inking of deep mastectomy margin. This is a modified radical mastectomy, with attached axillary contents. Prior to processing, the posterior margin is inked *black*. Note that the specimen has been washed and dried prior to cutting into it to avoid getting the ink on new cut surfaces.

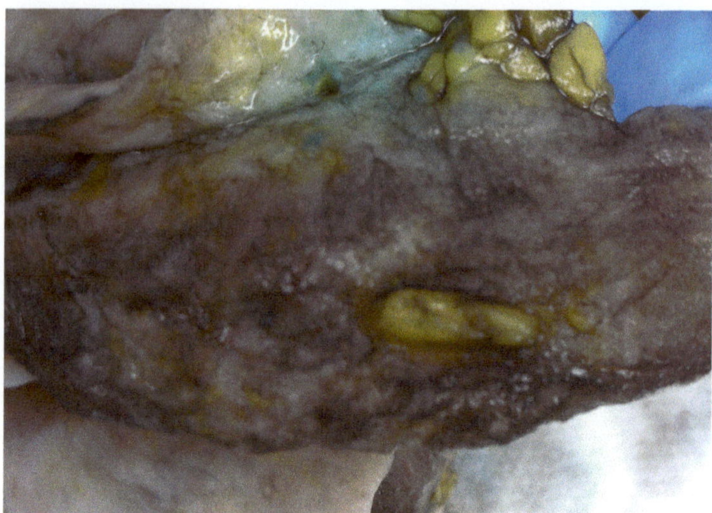

FIGURE 3.5 An example of ink seepage into the breast tissue. It is important to apply a mordant after inking the surgical margins. It is also a good idea to wash off excess ink and dry the surface, prior to slicing into it. The *black ink* is easy to see in histologic sections and this type of seepage can lead to difficulty in microscopic margin evaluation.

mapping protocol have raised concerns about exposure to radiation to personnel handling such specimens containing radioactive technitium. Immediate handling of such specimens may expose the pathologist or their assistants or trainees performing the gross examination to radioactivity, which may be an issue over long period of time. However, studies have suggested that such exposures are minimal. The established exposure limits for non-radiation workers is 500 mrem per year and typical exposure from sentinel node mapping is 1 mrem. Therefore, it is safe to handle these specimens in the gross room, though each laboratory should have specific policies and procedures for handling these specimens, in accordance with radiation safety and the state laws.

GROSS EXAMINATION OF THE SPECIMEN WITH A MASS

Breast tissue is mainly composed of fat with lesser percentage of fibrous tissue, in most cases. The tumors appear somewhat different depending upon the histologic type. Invasive ductal carcinoma is typically irregular in shape, often extending into

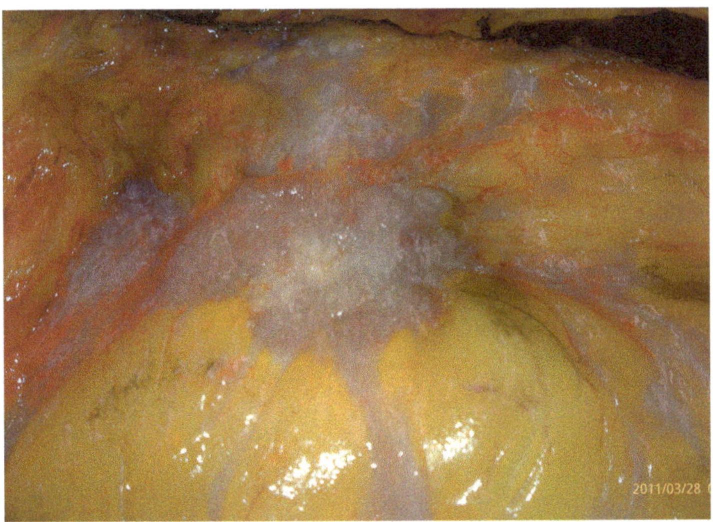

FIGURE 3.6 Invasive carcinoma involving the surgical margin. This tumor is homogeneous in appearance and extends into fibrous septa. It appears to merge into fibrous breast tissue, which is present at the *black-inked* deep margin. To the left, there is a biopsy site with a metal clip.

adipose tissue with long tentacles. It is firm, gray-white, and gritty to cut. The cut surface retracts unlike the surrounding benign breast tissue (Figs. 3.6–3.10).

Invasive lobular carcinoma may have an appearance similar to invasive ductal carcinoma. But quite often, it is more poorly circumscribed and less firm. It often cuts and feels like fibrous breast tissue. Its interface with the adjacent benign breast tissue is difficult to appreciate and is often better felt than seen (Figs. 3.11–3.13). Mucinous carcinoma is very distinct in appearance due to pools of mucin; however, this is a very uncommon type of breast cancer. Medullary carcinoma and its variants present with a rounded, fleshy mass with bulging cut surface. It can mimic a benign lesion.

Ductal carcinoma in situ mostly does not form a mass. However, some high-grade cases may appear as a vaguely defined, rubbery mass. The cut surfaces show the dilated ducts with punctate areas of necrosis.

The appearance of benign lesions is very different from the malignant lesions. Fibrocystic changes show pale white rubbery

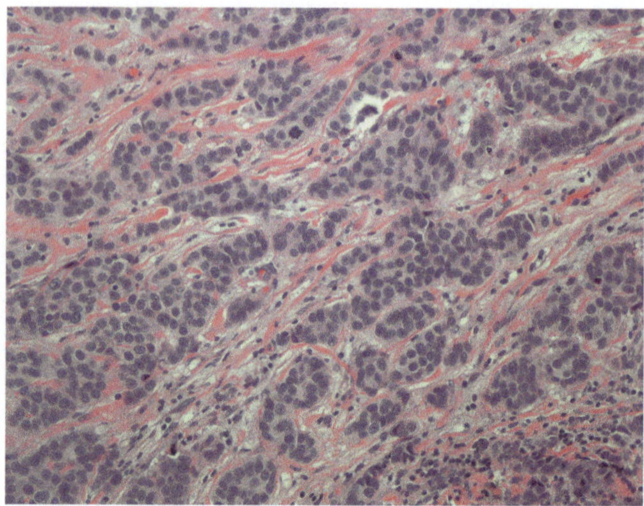

FIGURE 3.7 Invasive ductal carcinoma. Histologic section from the tumor in Fig. 3.6. This is an invasive ductal carcinoma, grade 2. Note the absence of gland formation, moderate nuclear pleomorphism, and mitotic activity.

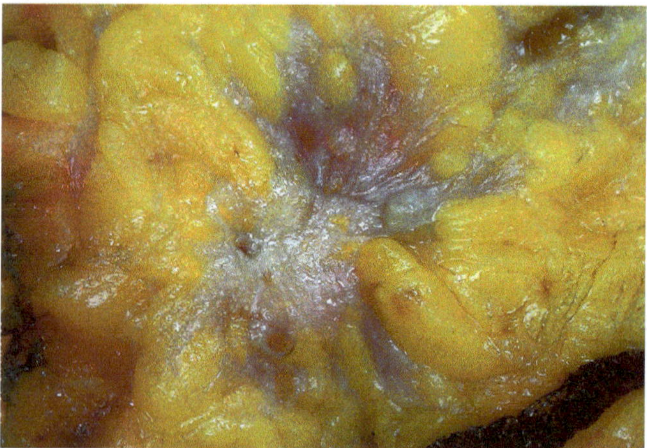

FIGURE 3.8 Typical gross appearance of an invasive ductal carcinoma. The tumor is gray-white, stellate, and infiltrates the fatty breast tissue. There is a small biopsy site at the left inferior part of the tumor mass. Also note the second, larger biopsy site is at the upper right corner of the image, away from the tumor.

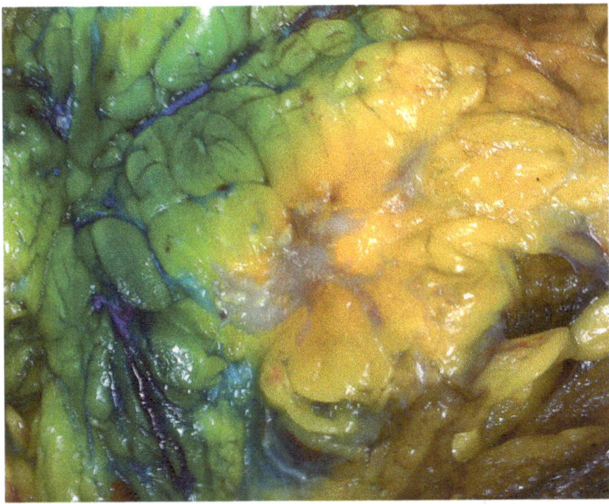

FIGURE 3.9 Small invasive cancer after SLN mapping. There is fat necrosis at the superior edge of the tumor mass, caused by the needle biopsy. To the left, the breast tissue contains methylene blue dye, injected during the sentinel lymph node mapping procedure.

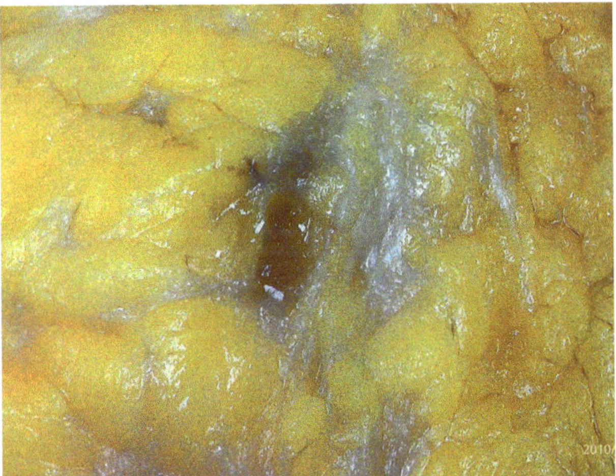

FIGURE 3.10 Invasive tumor with a biopsy cavity and biopsy site marker. An irregular tumor mass is seen in this image. Its borders are ill-defined and infiltrative. There is a biopsy site in the left half of the tumor and it contains a metal clip.

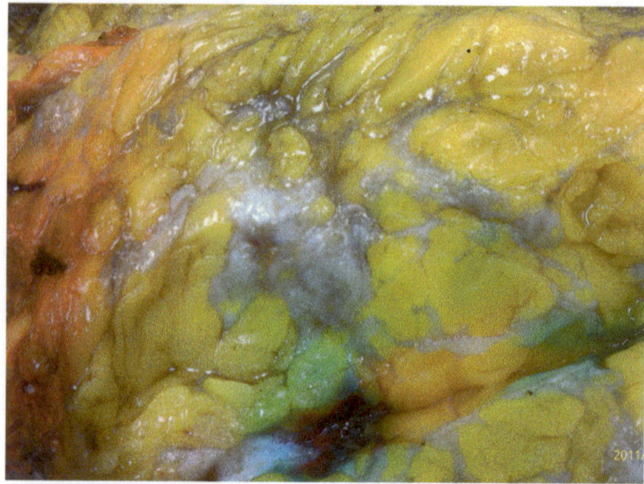

FIGURE 3.11 Gross appearance of invasive lobular carcinoma. The mass is easy to recognize, but it is pale white than typical invasive ductal carcinomas. Also note the multifocal nature of this tumor, which can be hard to identify, as it appears similar to benign fibrous breast tissue. There is a biopsy cavity at inferior edge of the tumor.

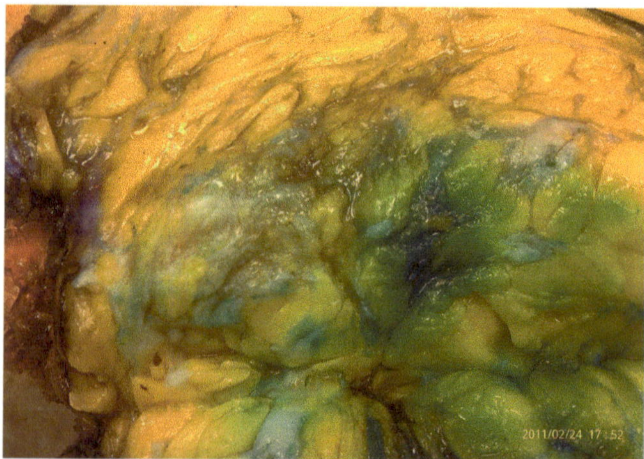

FIGURE 3.12 Gross appearance of invasive lobular carcinoma. This is a relatively difficult case on the basis of gross examination. The tumor is very poorly defined and resembles fibrocystic changes. It is in fact multifocal and bulges out on the surface, unlike invasive ductal carcinoma, which tends to retract after slicing. There is blue dye due to sentinel lymph mapping.

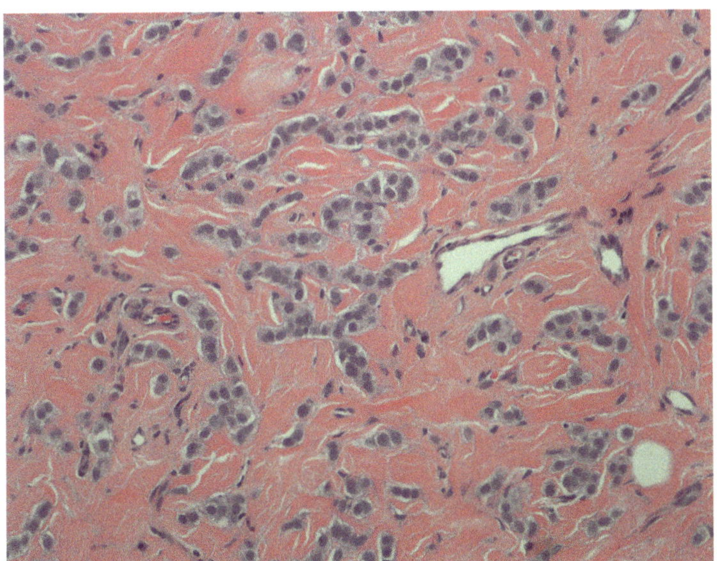

FIGURE 3.13 Invasive lobular carcinoma. Histologic section from the tumor in Figs. 3.11 and 3.12. This is an invasive lobular carcinoma. Note the single file and single cell growth pattern in the background of dense fibrous breast tissue.

tissue with light blue cysts. Fibroadenoma is often removed without much surrounding tissue. The lesion is white to light yellow with bulging cut surface. Phyllodes tumor may resemble a fibroadenoma, but in larger lesions, the leaf-like pattern can be appreciated.

The biopsy site should be identified in all cases. Imaging studies can aid in locating the biopsy site with ease. It appears as a hemorrhagic area, and a clip placed at the time of core needle biopsy must be identified (see Figs. 3.8–3.11). The biopsy cavity can sometimes be difficult to identify, if surgery was delayed for more than a few weeks. The appearance of the tumor can change a lot after neoadjuvant therapy. It can appear like untreated tumor in cases with no response to a vague area of dense fibrous tissue. In such cases, careful palpation can be more useful than visual examination alone (Figs. 3.14–3.18).

Axillary lymph nodes should be carefully dissected out to identify as many nodes as possible for microscopic evaluation. A minimum of ten nodes must be histologically examined for

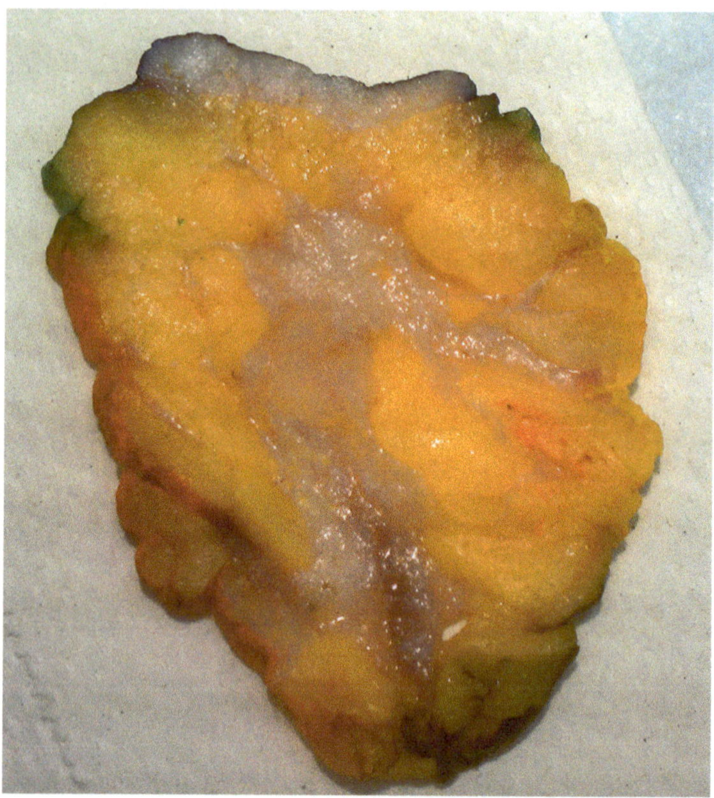

FIGURE 3.14 Nonresponding invasive ductal carcinoma after neoadjuvant therapy. This large tumor did not show any significant clinical response after treatment. This is a slice from a salvage lumpectomy. Tumor is 8 mm below the skin surface, extends deep into the breast and is close to the deep margin.

adequate nodal staging. Inspection, palpation, and attention to tissue around larger vessels help in performing the gross examination and identification of axillary lymph nodes (Fig. 3.19).

SAMPLING OF A BREAST MASS

The sectioning of palpable lesions is relatively straightforward. If the entire lesion or tumor has a relatively homogeneous gross appearance, then 3–4 sections are sufficient to capture all the necessary information. In general, it is a good idea so serially

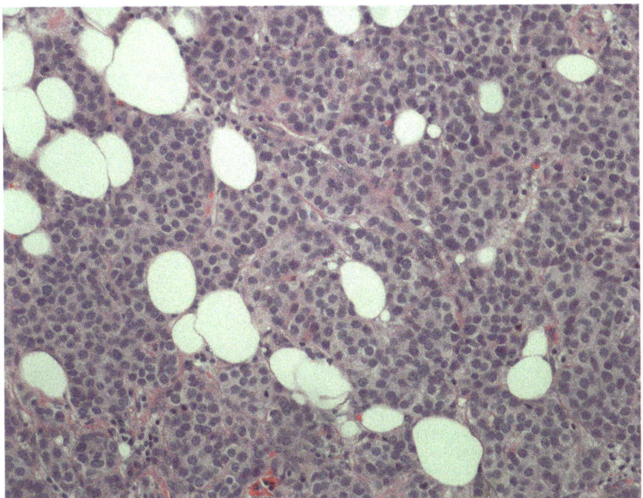

FIGURE 3.15 Residual tumor after neoadjuvant therapy. A higher power view of the tumor in Fig. 3.14. This invasive ductal carcinoma has a very irregular growth pattern and this can be seen here as the tumor cells infiltrate and surround the adipose tissue. This tumor failed to respond to neoadjuvant chemotherapy.

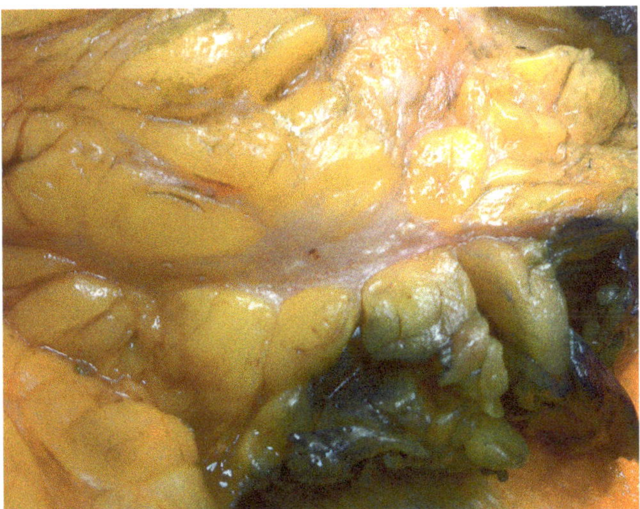

FIGURE 3.16 Gross appearance of the tumor bed after neoadjuvant therapy. This specimen is from a mastectomy after neoadjuvant chemotherapy. An irregular, stellate lesion with fibrous tissue, focal pinpoint hemorrhage, and possible foci of necrosis is seen, a few millimeters from the inked surgical margin.

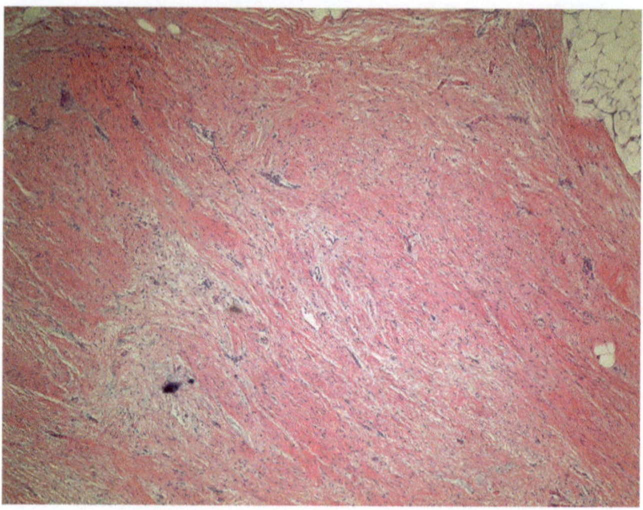

FIGURE 3.17 Tumor bed after neoadjuvant therapy. Histologic appearance of the area identified as tumor bed in Fig. 3.16. There is extensive fibrosis but no definite residual tumor cells can be identified.

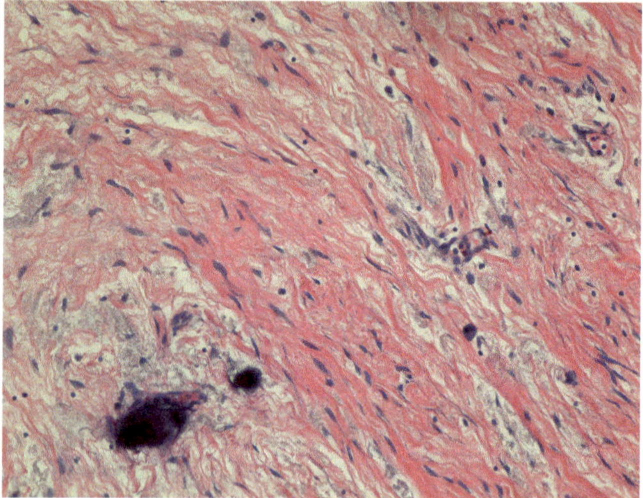

FIGURE 3.18 A high power view showing fibrosis and calcifications after neoadjuvant chemotherapy. A few capillaries, scattered lymphocytes, and rare mast cell are noted. No carcinoma is seen.

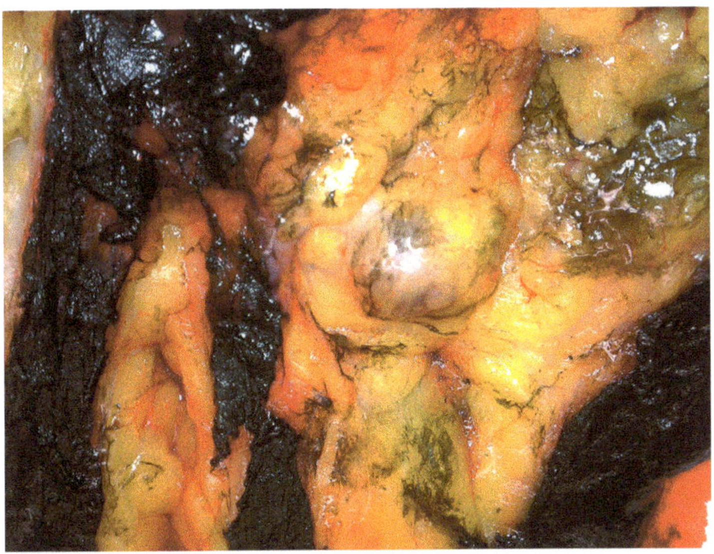

FIGURE 3.19 Identification of axillary lymph nodes. This is a closer view of the sliced mastectomy specimen seen in Figs. 3.3 and 3.4. This is the junction of upper outer quadrant and level I of axilla. There is a large, bulging positive axillary lymph node in this area.

submit the tumor in its longest dimension, provided the tumor mass is unifocal and less than 5 cm. At least one section should demonstrate the interface between the tumor and normal tissue. This section can be taken at the time of initial slicing of the specimen to start the tumor fixation time and may be used for predictive biomarker assessment, as it is likely to contain internal control tissue (discussed in more detail in Chap. 6). The rest of the sections should show the relationship of the tumor with the surrounding breast tissue. If the lesion is within 10 mm of any of the margins, then this relationship should be represented in specific sections. In case of totally fatty breast tissue around the tumor, sections to document grossly negative margins by more than 10 mm is neither necessary nor useful. Representative sections of uninvolved breast tissue should be included to document nonpalpable proliferative lesions. These sections should be taken from fibrous breast tissue, since it is unlikely to find any clinically useful lesion in pure adipose tissue. Such sections tend to process poorly, often leading to unnecessary expense of time and other resources. A study of

384 consecutive excisions performed for a palpable mass found that by focusing on fibrous tissue alone and submission of a maximum of ten cassettes after initial examination saved the expense of 18% of tissue block preparation and microscopic evaluation without missing any significant lesions. The rate of surgically significant lesions, such as atypical hyperplasias or carcinomas was 6.8% in their cohort. Only one case of atypical lobular hyperplasia was identified in sections from adipose tissue only. The authors recommended that additional sections be considered if the first ten blocks contain atypical hyperplasia or carcinoma. At least one section should include skin, if present. A detailed summary of cassettes should accompany the gross description to assist the pathologist performing the microscopic examination. Often a diagram to describe the topography of submitted sections is a very helpful aid.

Chapter 4
Handling of Specimens with a Nonpalpable Lesion

According to the American Cancer Society, about one in four cases diagnosed as breast cancer represent ductal carcinoma in situ (DCIS). The majority of these cases are nonpalpable. In addition, some small invasive tumors are only detected by imaging studies without forming a lump or a mass. For several years, frozen sections on excisions for nonpalpable lesions have been discouraged and intraoperative evaluation of these surgical specimens is no longer a standard practice. However, in 2009, the CAP has required a staging summary for DCIS that includes the documentation of extent of the disease and several other characteristics of this lesion. Therefore, the handling of breast specimens for nonpalpable lesions has become more critical (Fig. 4.1) and this chapter is dedicated to this subject.

CORRELATION WITH THE SPECIMEN RADIOGRAPH

The first step in processing excisions for nonpalpable lesions is to obtain specimen x-ray or digital image. Almost all such excisions have a needle/wire localization to guide the surgeon. Once the surgeon has finished the excision, a specimen radiograph is obtained (Figs. 4.2 and 4.3). This is transmitted to both the radiologist and the pathologist, either in the form of a film or a digital image. Once the radiologist confirms the complete removal of the imaging abnormality, this area is marked on the film or the image, the surgeon is notified and the pathology laboratory can proceed

S.K. Mohsin, *Frozen Section Library: Breast*, Frozen Section Library 9,
DOI 10.1007/978-1-4614-0718-8_4,

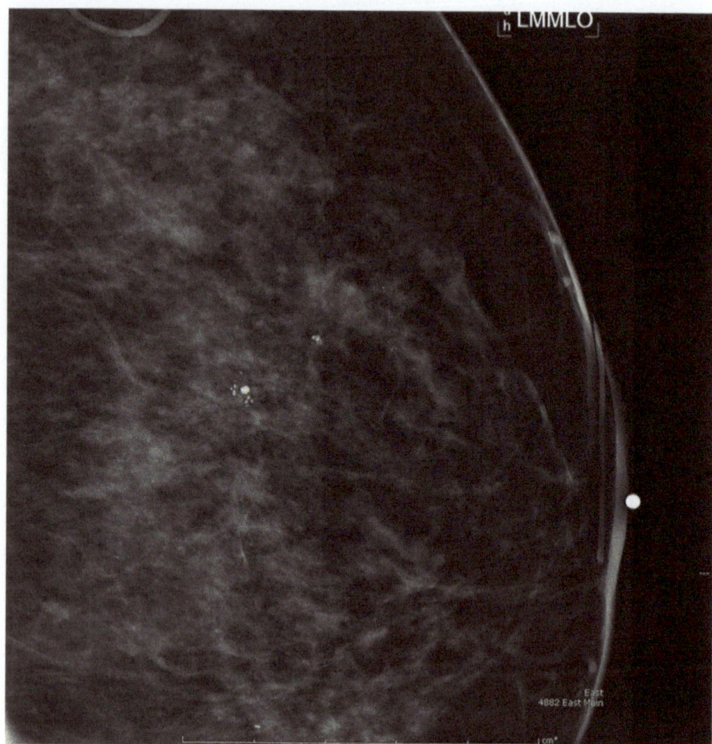

FIGURE 4.1 Diagnostic mammogram showing two clusters of calcifications. The one in central posterior location shows coarse calcifications and is considered benign. The anterior group is pleomorphic and fine and is classified indeterminate, prompting needle biopsy.

with the specimen processing. In certain institutions, the specimen radiograph is obtained either in the operative room or the pathology department. In these kinds of setup, the initial specimen handling is often done together by the surgeon, pathologist, and radiologist. Additional images of the sliced specimen may be taken to help the pathologist focus on the part of the specimen most likely to contain the area of interest. This may also help in selecting tissue for possible intraoperative evaluation, such as for close margins. During these steps, the pathologist gets to learn more details about the reason for excision and performs the correlation between the findings on corresponding imaging study and the specimen.

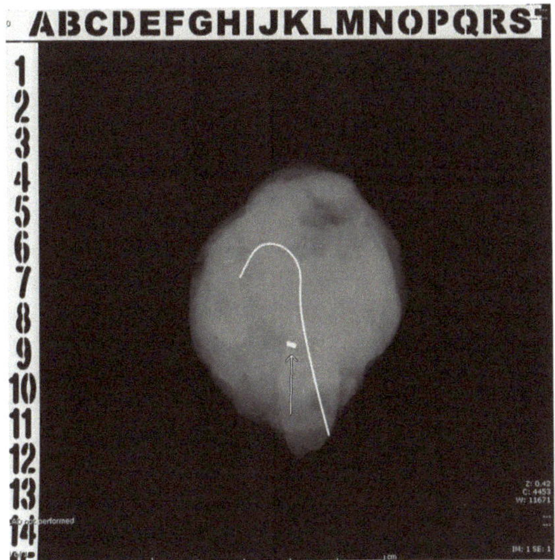

FIGURE 4.2 Specimen radiograph after needle localization. The specimen is placed on a radioopaque spec board. The wire hook is relatively away from the clip (*arrow*). There is a cluster of calcifications to the *right* of the *arrow*.

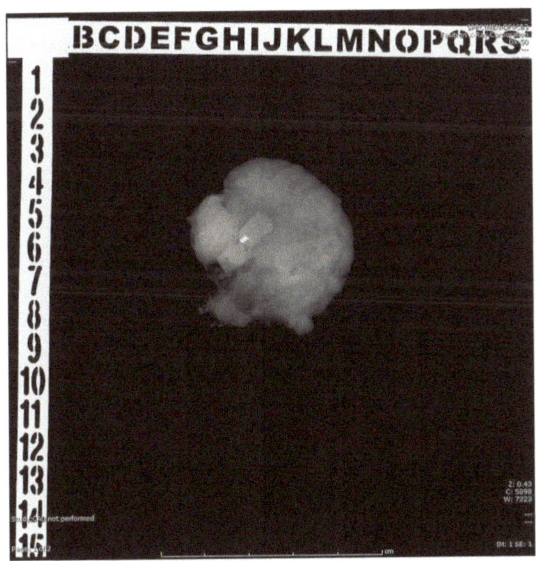

FIGURE 4.3 Specimen radiograph for a mass lesion. The mass appears as a rounded density at G 5/6 coordinates of the grid. There is a spiral metal clip next to the mass. Two rectangular radioopaque densities are due to markers placed on top of the specimen to mark the clip location.

PREPARATION OF THE SPECIMEN FOR PROCESSING

As stated in Chap. 3, the specimen should be weighed and measured in three dimensions. The area of radiologic abnormality should be marked on the surface of the specimen, corresponding to the area marked by the radiologist on the specimen radiograph. After that, the margins should be inked, using multiple inks (Figs. 4.4 and 4.5). After these steps, the specimen can be serially sectioned into 3–5-mm thick slices (Fig. 4.6). It is often difficult to cut fatty specimens into such thin slices at room temperature. The method described below can be a useful adjunct.

This method was developed and optimized in our laboratory and it allows sectioning of fatty breast tissue into thin slices without lengthy formalin fixation. The specimen is rapidly cooled on the surface by direct immersion in an isopentane bath at – 65°C for 5–60 s, based on size of the specimen. This makes the adipose tissue firm for a short time, allowing one to slice the specimen into 3–4-mm thick sections (Fig. 4.7). After examination, the tissue is placed in 10% NBF for tissue fixation. This method has been shown not to affect the histology or special stains including immunohistochemical stains.

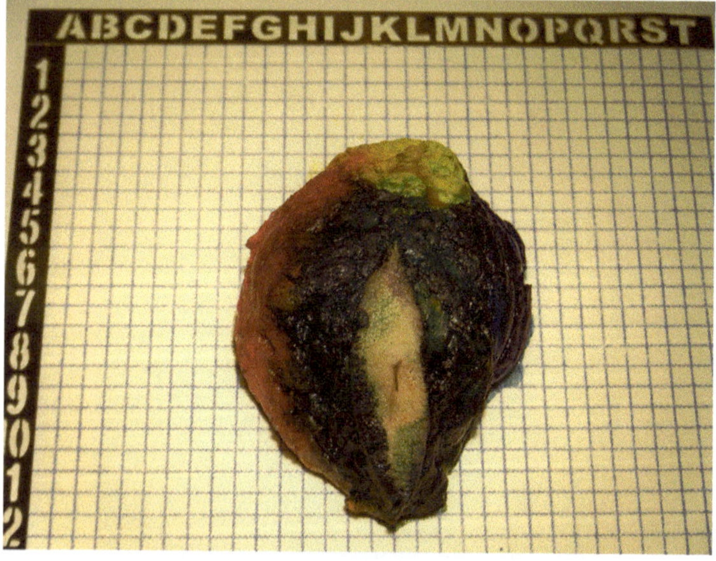

FIGURE 4.4 Wire-guided excision received on a spec board. The specimen radiograph was taken and showed the lesion at 4-5/H-J coordinates of the grid. The specimen margins have been inked using the protocol described in the text. The *red ink* marks the area of localization.

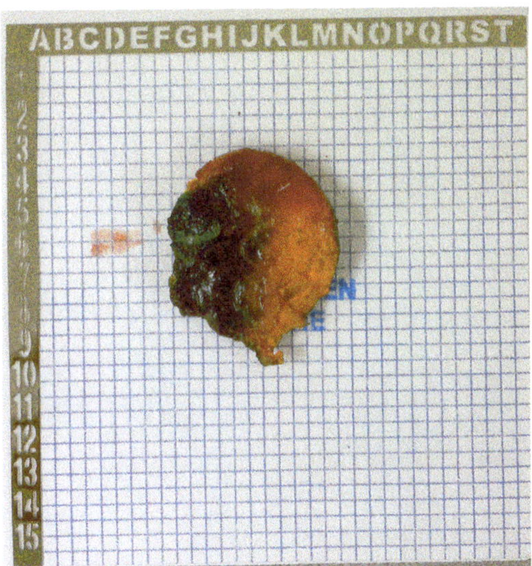

FIGURE 4.5 Inked specimen from needle localization. The surgeon has inked the specimen in the operating room using a sterile tissue inking kit and then placed it on the spec board for radiography (see Fig. 4.2). The *purple ink* (*center*) marks the area of the clip. The lesion is on the anterior margin (*green ink*). This case was a phyllodes tumor that required re-excision of this margin.

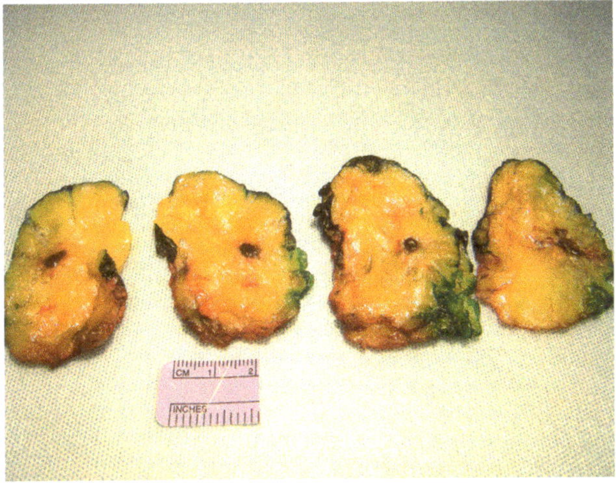

FIGURE 4.6 Specimen serially sectioned using standard method. These slices are 7–8-mm thick. It is difficult to cut thinner slices when breast tissue is so fatty. It allows for a good gross examination, showing a long biopsy cavity spanning four slices. However, the tissue needs to be trimmed for submitting sections for histology.

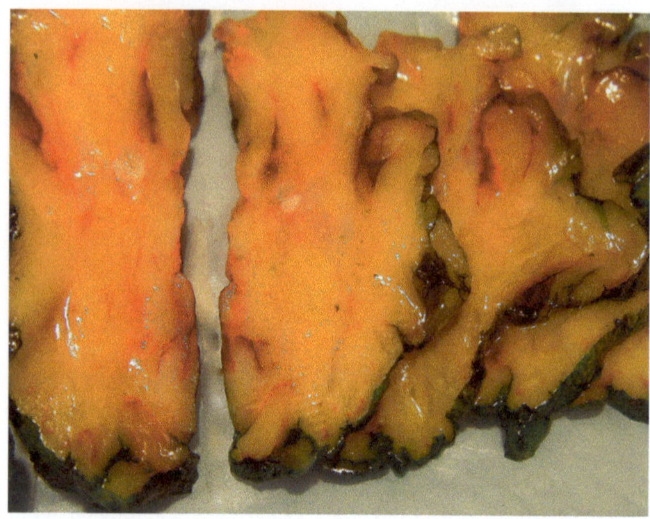

FIGURE 4.7 Specimen serially sectioned after gently freezing the surface. After this technique, it is possible to slice fatty breast tissue at 3-mm thick slices. In this case, the biopsy site contains pale white pellets. The tissue to the right of biopsy site is pink and vaguely nodular, representing high grade DCIS.

SAMPLING OF SPECIMEN WITH A NONPALPABLE LESION

The area of abnormality or lesion should be described using appropriate phrases for size in three dimensions, color, edges, feel of the cut-surface, and exact distance from all the margins (Figs. 4.6–4.9). The goal is to provide all the necessary sections to verify the findings of the gross examination and to assess all the microscopic characteristics of the lesion. In the majority of cases, selective or representative tissue sections should be submitted in a logical and methodical, yet cost-effective manner.

Some experts recommend submitting the entire specimen removed for a nonpalpable abnormality for microscopic evaluation. The reason behind this approach is to identify all premalignant lesions, which cannot be seen on gross examination. In the current environment of cost savings in delivering quality healthcare, these two seemingly contrary objectives require more thoughtful and evidence-based practice. The radiologically guided specimens can be handled in a fashion similar to lumpectomies. As described above, a clip or residual calcifications in the specimen radiograph identify the area of abnormality (Fig. 4.10). This can be marked on the surface of the specimen by a specific ink.

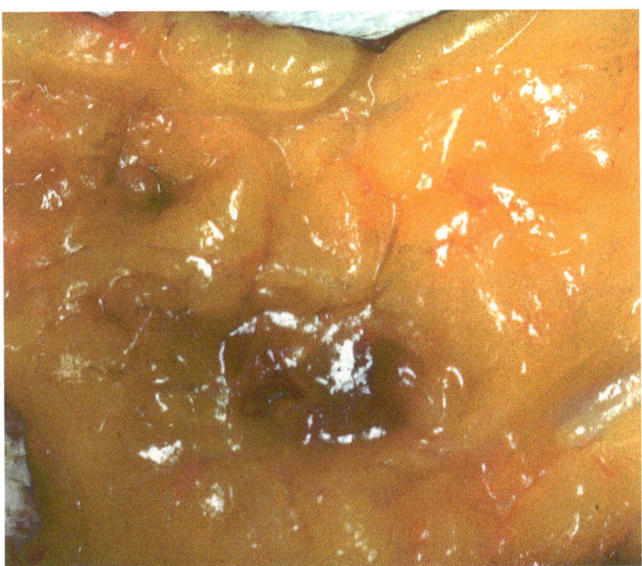

FIGURE 4.8 Close-up view of a biopsy cavity. There is focal organized hemorrhage and some fat necrosis. It is difficult to identify a specific lesion.

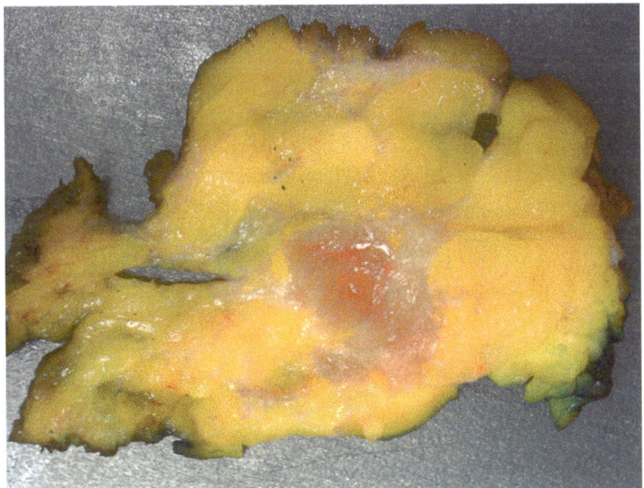

FIGURE 4.9 Biopsy site with a grossly identified otherwise nonpalpable lesion. This nonpalpable lesion is relatively obvious after slicing. Its margins are poorly demarcated and the center shows blood due to recent needle biopsy.

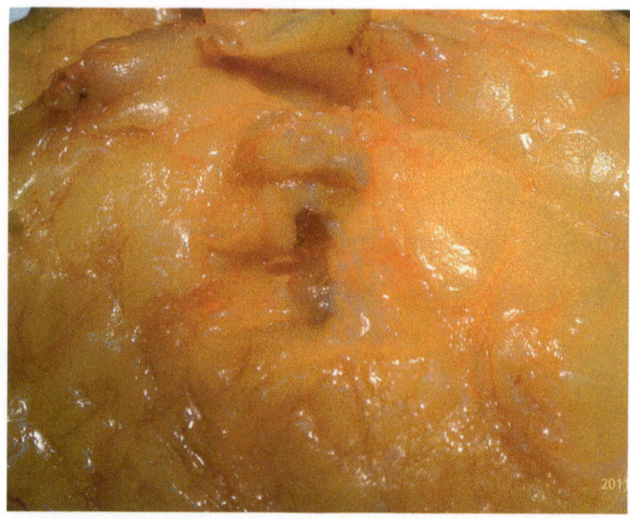

FIGURE 4.10 Biopsy site with a clip. This small biopsy cavity contains a coiled metallic clip. The specimen is fatty with no obvious lesion.

Once the specimen has been serially sectioned, the biopsy cavity or a scar with the clip serves as the area of localization. The specimen can then be treated as a lumpectomy and thoroughly sampled. The tissue taken for microscopic evaluation should include the entire area of radiographic lesion with focus on the relationship with surrounding breast tissue and surgical margins. In some cases, the area of localization is still obscure and radiographs of the sliced specimen can be helpful in directing to the area of concern.

The CAP recommends the use of tumor summary for reporting cases with DCIS without invasive cancer. The current version of the tumor summary for DCIS requires accurate estimate of the extent of DCIS. This includes information obtained from the gross and microscopic examination. The method described above for processing wire-guided excisions can help achieve consistent protocols that can meet the requirements for gross examination of cases with radiologically detected DCIS. A diagram with details regarding the areas that are submitted in each cassette is required to meet the recommendations. Either a handdrawn diagram or specimen radiograph of all the slices of the specimen may be used to mark the places from where the sections are taken. Using either method, the pathologist examining the slides can identify the number of slices involved with DCIS and calculate the extent of DCIS.

Chapter 5
Core Needle Biopsies

Percutaneous core needle biopsies comprise the most common type of breast specimens in current practice. The indications for such biopsies include palpable and nonpalpable breast lesions. The majority of these biopsies are performed with the aid of imaging modalities, such as mammogram, ultrasound, or MRI (Figs. 5.1 and 5.2). The operator is usually a breast radiologist or a surgeon. Neither sample adequacy check nor diagnostic evaluation is requested on such samples. However, documentation of certain pertinent information at the time of gross examination is critical for the reasons provided below. It is therefore important that the handling of this sample is discussed separately in this book.

The gross evaluation of core needle biopsies is very simple and similar to other small biopsy specimens. However, the final pathology report on these samples cannot be reliably completed in the current standard of practice without certain pieces of information. The pathology report on these samples requires correlation with findings on imaging studies that triggered the biopsy, in addition to the clinical presentation and clinical breast examination. The physician who performs the biopsy is responsible for the final correlation. The CAP and the American Society of Clinical Oncology (ASCO) guidelines recommend using these core biopsies for the assessment of predictive biomarkers, if the sample contains breast carcinoma. In order to comply with this recommendation, core biopsy samples are subjected to time to fixation and fixation length stipulations (see more details in Chap. 6).

S.K. Mohsin, *Frozen Section Library: Breast*, Frozen Section Library 9,
DOI 10.1007/978-1-4614-0718-8_5,

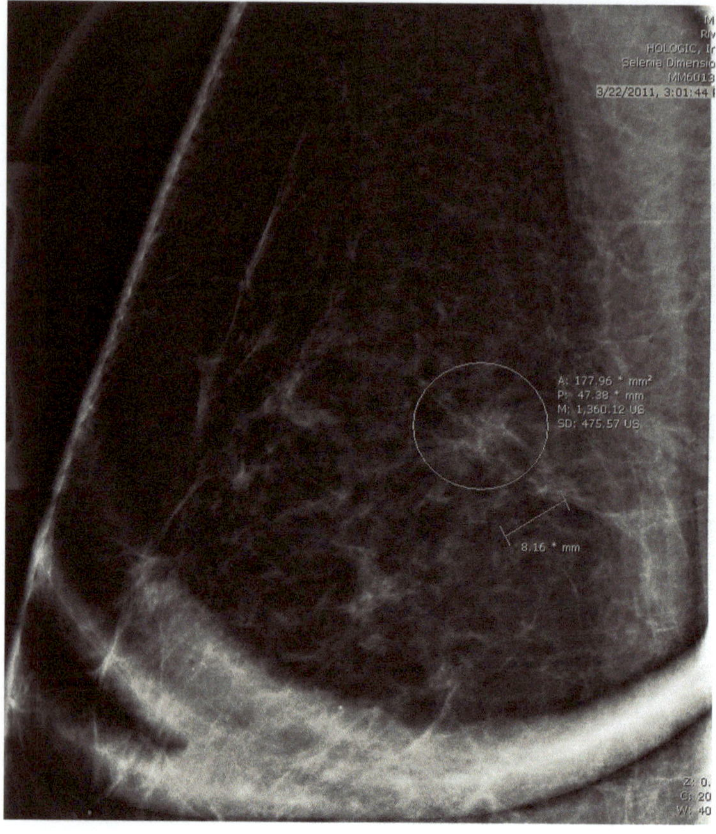

FIGURE 5.1 Mammogram with a spiculated mass. This diagnostic mammogram shows a discrete, spiculated density measuring 8 mm, characteristic of invasive cancer.

RADIOLOGIC–PATHOLOGIC CORRELATION

A radiologist typically performs the biopsies triggered by an abnormal mammogram. The indications include mass, density, distortion, and calcifications. The most important initial step is to get all the necessary information about the clinical examination and imaging studies so that the pathologist can document the information required to perform radiologic–pathologic correlation. This is best accomplished at the time of specimen accession and gross examination. It may be useful to aid the physicians to collect and document all the useful clinical information on the pathology requisition. A sticker or preprinted area on the specimen requisition can help remind the submitting physician to provide relevant

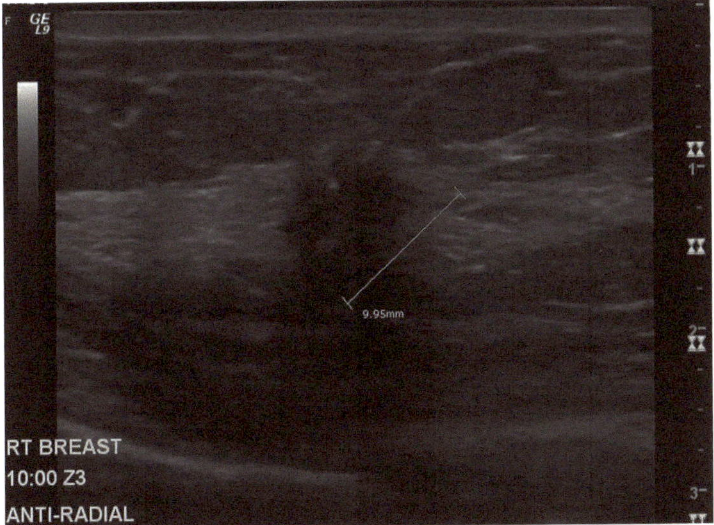

FIGURE 5.2 Breast ultrasound with a hypoechoic mass. This focused ultrasound of the density shown in Fig. 5.1 confirms an irregular mass with shadowing, characteristic of invasive cancer. The tumor was measured to be almost 10 mm by this method.

TABLE 5.1 A template like this embedded in the specimen requisition form assists the submitting physician to record useful clinical and radiologic information for the pathologist.

Specimen laterality: Right or Left	*Location*: o'clock
Distance from the nipple: _____cm	*Type of lesion*: Mass/density/distortion
BIRADS classification:	*Size of the lesion*: _____cm

clinical information and the indication for the biopsy (Table 5.1). The best way to get the physicians and their staff to fill these out is by educating them about the importance of this information to generate the report that meets their expectations allowing them to perform the final clinicopathologic correlation.

GROSS EXAMINATION OF CORE BIOPSIES

For stereotactic biopsies performed for calcifications, the radiologists typically x-rays the cores to make sure the calcifications are present in the removed tissue. The radiologists then have different options to draw pathologist's attention to the core identified as harboring the calcifications (Figs. 5.3 and 5.4). The cores may be placed in a separate specimen container, which is labeled as

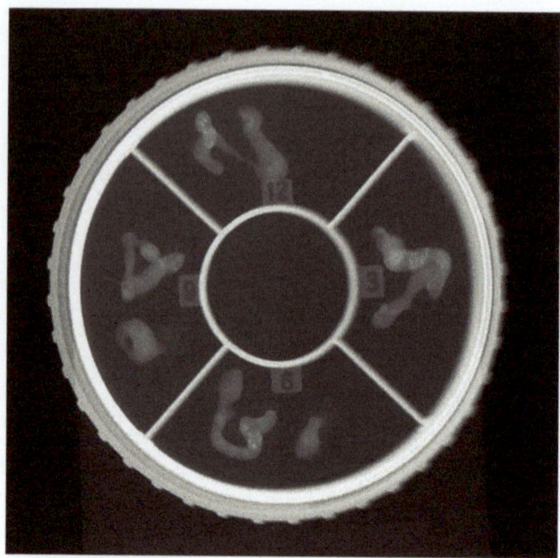

Figure 5.3 One of the methods to segregate cores containing calcifications. After removing the cores for calcifications on the mammogram, the radiologist images the core. This is one of the methods where the cores are separated into a specific chamber to identify the ones with the calcifications. Note a cluster of calcifications in the cores present in 3 and 6 o'clock compartments.

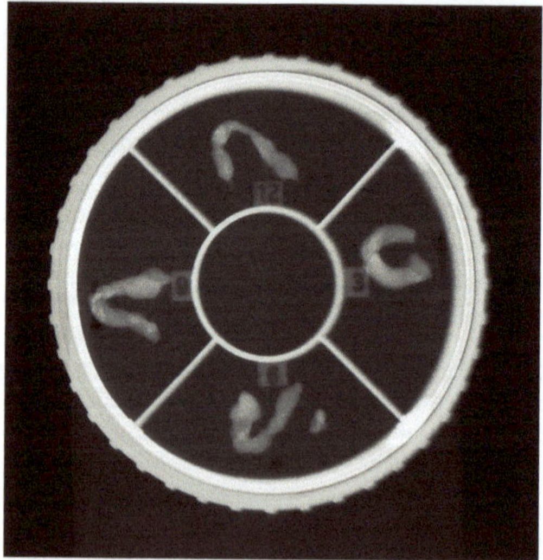

Figure 5.4 Radiograph of the breast cores for a mass. The cores with the mass, which appear as gray-white areas versus yellow fat, are in 3 and 6 o'clock compartments.

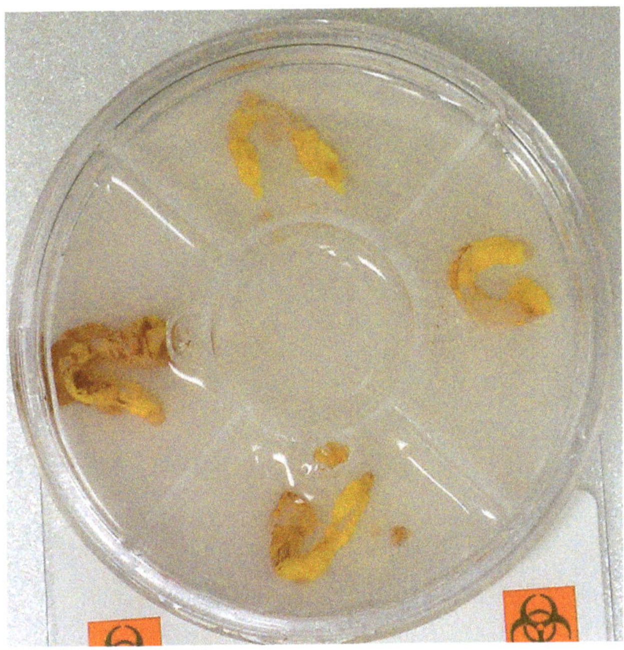

FIGURE 5.5 Breast cores done under mammographic guidance. The petri-dish-like plastic container is shown here containing cores with the lesion in separate compartments (see Fig. 5.4). Such cores are submitted in designated tissue cassettes and undergo additional H&E sections to ensure identification of the lesion.

"cores with calcifications" or they may be placed in a tissue cassette, which is itself placed in the specimen container. Some places use petri-dish-like containers with several compartments and may place the cores containing the lesion in a specific chamber (Fig. 5.5).

The gross examination should state that a specimen radiograph is available. The cores should be counted and measured, along with their nature as fatty or fibrous (Fig. 5.6). It is useful to document the number of cores submitted in each cassette. The tissue cassettes containing the targeted cores should be clearly identified in the gross description of the specimen. These steps help the pathologist performing the microscopic evaluation. It is the responsibility of the pathologist issuing the report on these specimens to document the histologic findings that correspond to the lesion seen on the imaging study (Figs. 5.7 and 5.8).

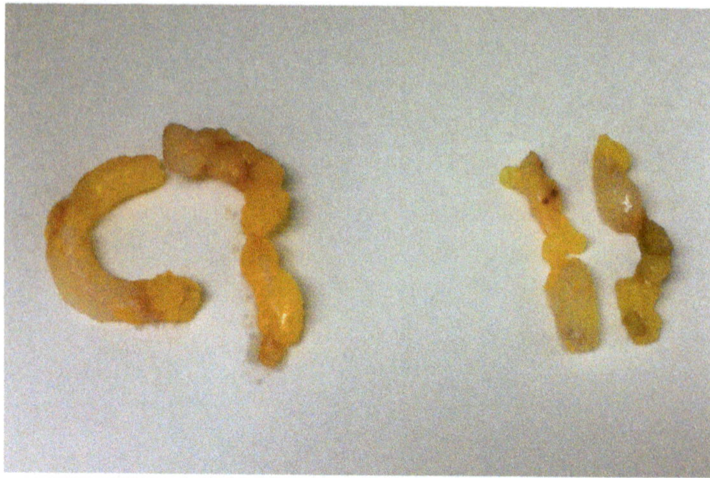

FIGURE 5.6 Gross appearance of breast cores. These cores were obtained using 11-gauge biopsy needles. The two cores on the *left* are from the area of mass lesion obtained by stereotactic method (seen in Figs. 5.4 and 5.5). The other two cores were obtained using ultrasound guidance.

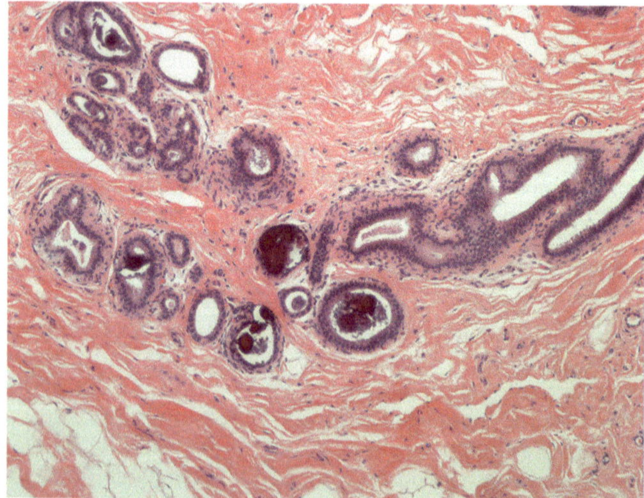

FIGURE 5.7 Core biopsy performed to evaluate calcifications. This is the histologic finding and correlation to the radiograph shown in Fig. 5.3. The microcalcifications are associated with columnar cell lesion of breast.

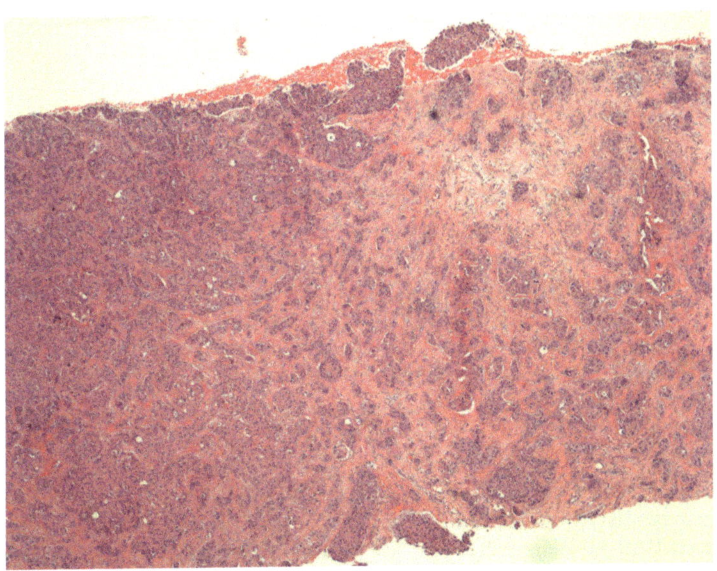

FIGURE 5.8 Core biopsy performed to evaluate a mass. This sample was obtained to assess a suspicious mass on mammogram and ultrasound. It shows a high-grade invasive ductal carcinoma, correlating to the mass seen in the imaging studies.

TISSUE PROCESSING OF BREAST CORES

The use of large gauge needles during stereotactic-guided core biopsies results in relatively thick specimens, which can be quite fatty. It is not a good idea to process these kinds of breast biopsies with other biopsy samples, such as GI or skin biopsies. In fact, some of the biopsies samples obtained in this fashion can be up to 3-mm in diameter, which pushes the limits of tissue thickness that can be optimally processed in the biopsy cycle of conventional and any cycle of the microwave tissue processors (see Fig. 5.6). Some of these samples may need to be sliced in half to bring the thickness to within the recommended limits.

MICROTOMY GUIDELINES FOR BREAST CORES

It is important to create and follow specific microtomy protocols for these needle biopsy specimens. These guidelines for the histotechnologist are typically captured on the tissue cassettes. This can be accomplished by a variety of methods, such as placing a preprinted paper in the cassette with instructions about the number and sequence of tissue section levels. This information can be printed on the cassette directly from the laboratory information system or by using barcodes. Most laboratories follow the published guidelines while some develop their own methods to cut enough sections for H&E stained slides to ensure the lesion is represented in histologic sections, minimizing recuts, and delays. This is especially true for the core needle biopsies performed for calcifications. For such specimens, the laboratory may chose to obtain additional sections upfront on cores shown by specimen radiograph to contain the calcifications. All these pieces of information need to be captured at the time of gross examination and documented in the gross description.

The objective of the microscopic examination of the cores is to identify the histologic changes that explain the radiologic findings. To achieve this goal, pathology laboratories use different protocols for sectioning the tissue blocks. It is difficult to recommend a specific method; however, these basic principles should be kept in mind. First, care should be taken at the time of embedding tissue specimen in paraffin block to ensure all the cores are separated (nonoverlapping) and are in a single plane for microtomy. Second, the block should be gently trimmed and then leveled to provide histologic sections from different depths of the cores for histologic evaluation. Third, ideally a fixed protocol of 4–5 H&E levels, at least 25–50 microns apart should be prepared. Fourth, the interpreting pathologist should review all the available information, including radiology reports at the time of microscopic examination, in order to issue a comprehensive pathology report.

Breast ultrasound is the most common way to further characterize the nature of a density or mass identified on mammogram. Ultrasound-guided biopsies are much easier to perform and are currently the method of choice to sample both the solid as well as complex cystic lesions. On the other hand, MRI-guided biopsies are relatively difficult and more time consuming to perform and are reserved for lesions seen only on the MRI and cannot be located by the second look, focused ultrasound of the area. Again, the pieces of information required to assess these types of core needle biopsies are the same as those for stereotactic biopsies.

Finally, the time to fixation and fixation duration needs to be recorded in the pathology report. This information is only needed if the diagnosis of malignancy is made on core needle biopsy. However, from a practical point of view, it is not possible to ask the gross room staff to make a judgment to record this information in selected cases. Therefore, it is a good idea to capture this information on all types of breast specimens. These requirements are discussed in the next chapter.

Chapter 6

Regulatory Requirements for Breast Specimens

Several aspects of breast pathology are affected by either regulatory requirements or recommendations and standards, to which the laboratory must comply in order to maintain accreditation as a licensed laboratory or an accredited breast program. For the rest of this chapter, these requirements or recommendations are lumped together as standards, which need to be documented in either laboratory files or patient reports. From the point of view of workflow, these standards affect preanalytic and analytic variables.

CURRENT STANDARDS FOR TISSUE FIXATION

The CAP and ASCO have set standards for the initial handling of certain types of breast specimens and compliance with these standards is required for accreditation. The clinical practice standard of assessing predictive biomarkers in newly diagnosed invasive breast cancers and at least estrogen receptor in DCIS is well established. The new requirements apply to all such breast samples that contain either DCIS or invasive breast cancer. Though the laboratories may decide to assess these biomarkers either in the diagnostic needle biopsies or the final surgical specimen, from a practical point of view, nearly all breast specimens fall under this category with rare exceptions, such as inflammatory lesions and a few other types of breast surgical specimens. These standards require documentation of two critical time periods, which have been recognized to affect the results of predictive biomarkers, i.e., estrogen receptor (ER), progesterone receptor (PR), and human epidermal growth factor receptor 2 (HER2). *Time to fixation*

S.K. Mohsin, *Frozen Section Library: Breast*, Frozen Section Library 9,
DOI 10.1007/978-1-4614-0718-8_6,

(cold ischemia time) for the tumor is defined as the time interval between loss of vascular supply to the tumor until it is exposed to a fixative such as 10% neutral-buffered formalin (NBF). Prolonged ischemia can lead to degradation of these proteins and thus false-negative results. The optimal cold ischemia time for breast tumors has been set to less than 60 min. *Fixation duration* is the time from exposure of the tumor to 10% NBF until the tumor enters the steps of processing with alcohols or other similar chemicals. Both shorter and prolonged tissue fixation can contribute to false-negative and false-positive predictive factor results. The optimal fixation duration is currently set between 6 and 72 h for ER and PR and 6–48 h for HER2. These time points encompass areas both outside and in the pathology laboratory. Therefore, the task of meeting these standards is much more difficult for the pathology laboratory, which performs and reports these tests.

EFFECTS OF SUBOPTIMAL TISSUE FIXATION

The effect of improper fixation and processing can be seen on routine H&E sections. These include cytoplasmic vacuolation and loss, retraction from adjacent cells and stroma, gradual loss of nuclear details, pyknosis and fragmentation, and inability to count the mitotic figures (Table 6.1 and Figs. 6.1–6.7). However, by the time such changes are appreciated, the cells of interest can often be severely damaged at the protein and nucleic acid level, making the assessment of biomarkers very difficult or impossible (Fig. 6.8). Both the nuclear and membrane bound proteins, such as ER and HER2 show progressive loss of staining due to lack of fixation (Figs. 6.9–6.15). Tissues processed too quickly, without the minimum 6–8 h of formalin fixation are at risk for exposure to alcohol-based solutions in the tissue processor. This can lead to false-positive results because the immunohistochemical assays

TABLE 6.1 Effects of improper fixation of tissue on morphologic features of the tumor cells.

- Both the nuclear and cytoplasm shows changes and the relationship of the tumor cells with the surrounding stroma is altered.
- There is cellular edema with retraction of cytoplasmic membrane, likely due to loss of adhesion molecules.
- Initially the cytoplasm appears vacuolated, followed by loss of organelles, which appears as loss of pink, granular cytoplasm.
- The nuclear details are lost first, such as nucleolus, followed by pyknosis and fragmentation of nucleus mimicking apoptosis.
- At the end, only a generalized basophilia is left where the epithelial cells were located.

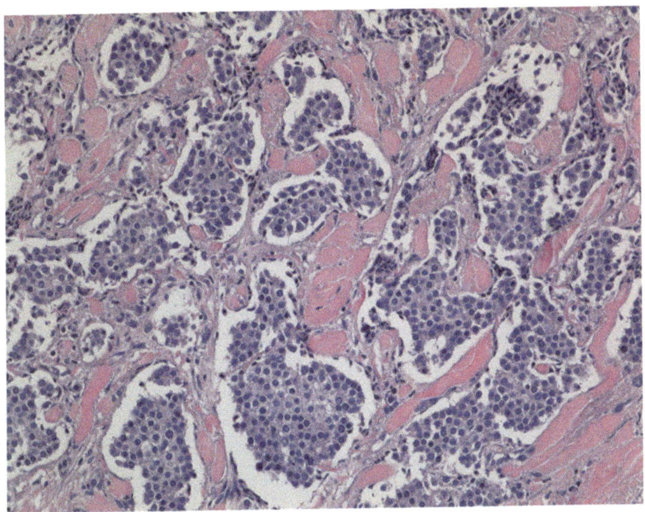

FIGURE 6.1 Early changes due to delayed tissue fixation. There is mild cellular edema and retraction of tumor clusters from the surrounding stroma. The individual tumor cells appear relatively preserved in nuclear and cytoplasmic details.

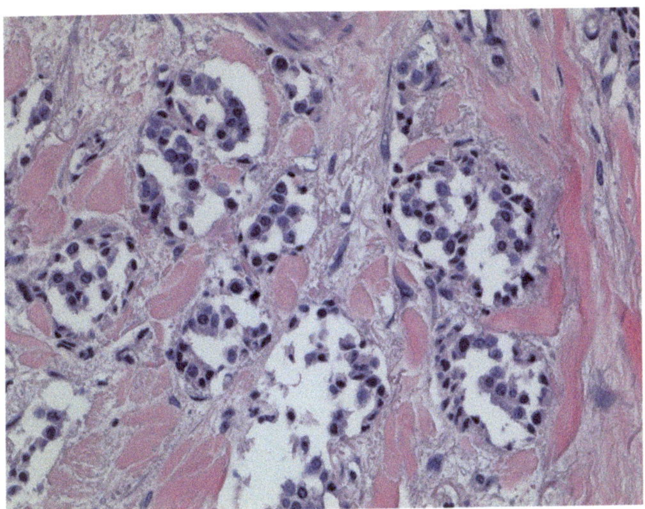

FIGURE 6.2 Advanced changes due to lack of adequate tissue fixation. There is marked cellular edema, separation of tumor cells from the surrounding stroma, and breakdown of intercellular adhesion with partial loss of cytoplasm.

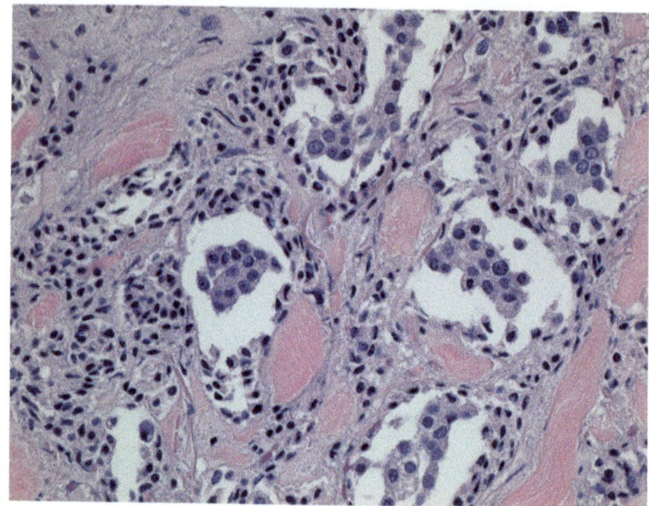

FIGURE 6.3 Heterogeneity in effects of inadequate fixation. The degree and extent of autolysis are unpredictable in breast tumors. Here, one can see some tumor cells with minimal cytologic changes, next to tumor cells with marked loss of nuclear and cytoplasmic details.

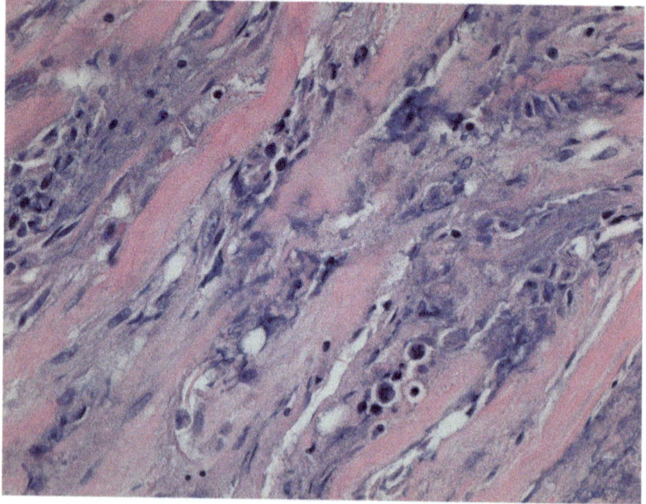

FIGURE 6.4 Changes seen at very advanced stage of cellular degeneration due to lack of fixation. The cellular structures can no longer be recognized. A few membrane bound structures containing nuclear debris can be seen.

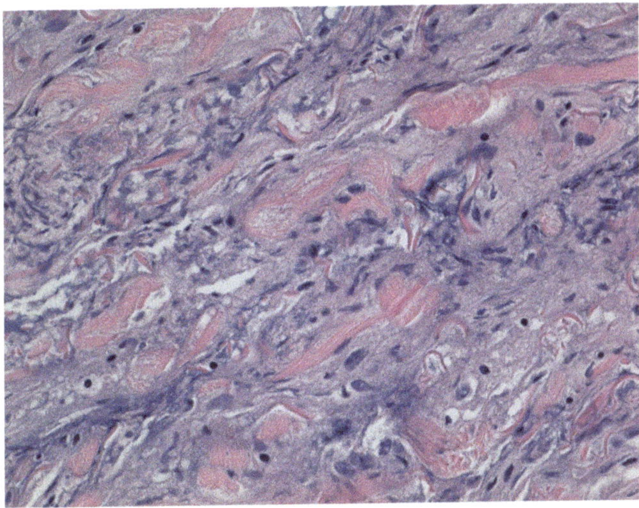

FIGURE 6.5 Endstage tissue loss due to inadequate fixation. The tumor cells have autolyzed leaving a generalized pale chromasia. No cellular details can be recognized.

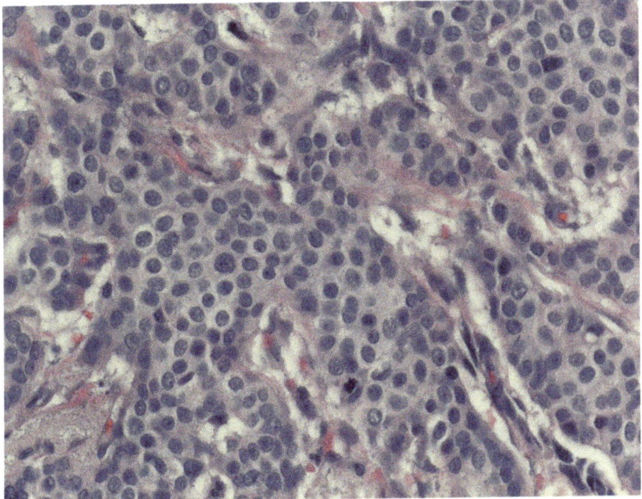

FIGURE 6.6 Optimally fixed grade 2 invasive ductal carcinoma. This well-fixed tissue displays great cytoplasmic and nuclear details, such as variable chromatin. The tumor cells adhere to each other and also appear attached to the surround stroma (compare to Figs. 6.1–6.5).

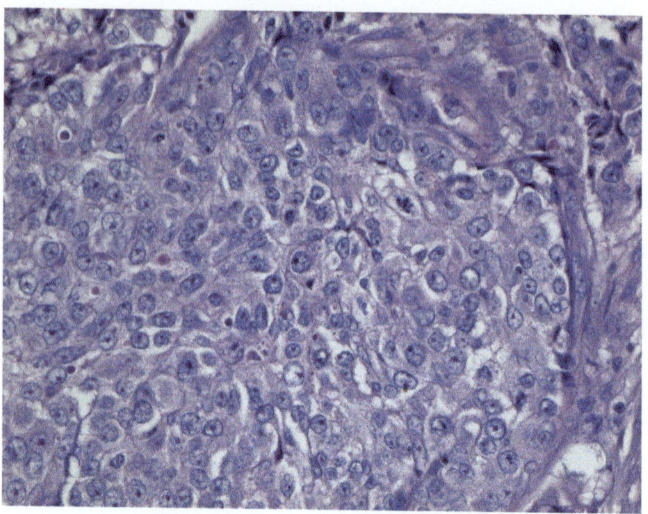

FIGURE 6.7 An example of adequately fixed high-grade tumor. This well-fixed invasive ductal carcinoma shows nuclear details, which are critical in determining the histologic grade. For example, the chromatin pattern, nucleoli, and mitotic figures are easy to evaluate.

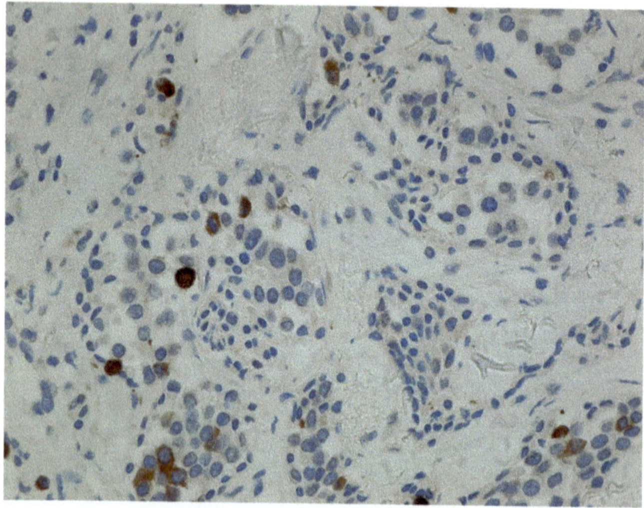

FIGURE 6.8 An example of loss of key proteins due to improper fixation. In this case, the morphological features are still somewhat intact, but cytokeratin 7 is lost in most of the tumor cells. In general, cytokeratin stains are fairly robust and work in poorly preserved tissues. In breast tumors, this is not the case and therefore, negative immunostains should be interpreted with caution.

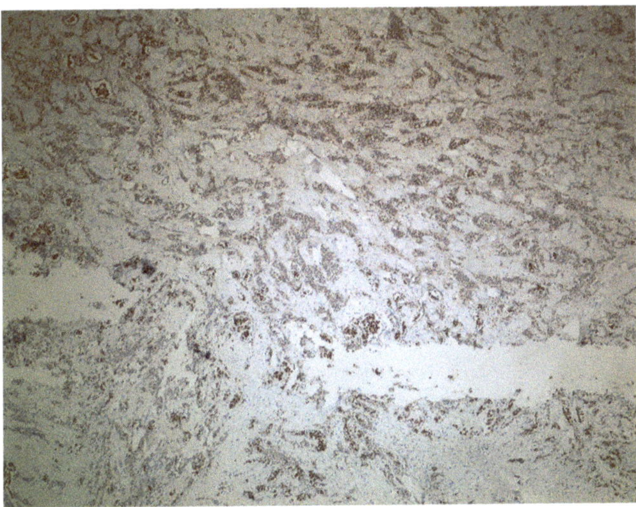

FIGURE 6.9 Heterogeneity in ER staining in a poorly preserved tumor. Despite significant loss of ER protein in this case, ER can be interpreted as positive, though the exact semiquantitative interpretation is not possible.

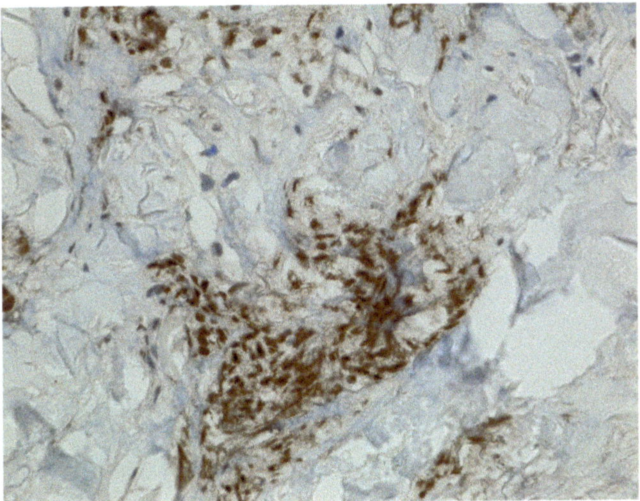

FIGURE 6.10 Progressive loss of ER staining in suboptimally fixed tissue. This part of the tumor shows cytolysis. The cellular and nuclear details are lost. ER staining is seen as a blush but it is uninterpretable.

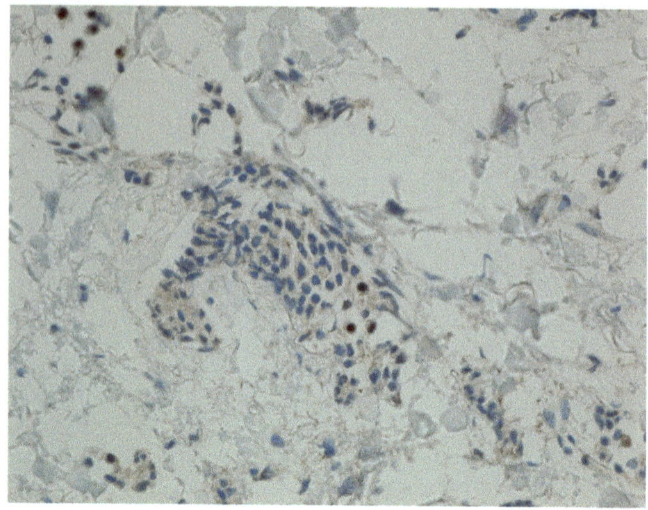

FIGURE 6.11 Loss of ER protein due to lack of fixation. An example of breast cancer with delayed tissue fixation. In this case, tumor morphology is partly intact but ER staining is almost completely lost.

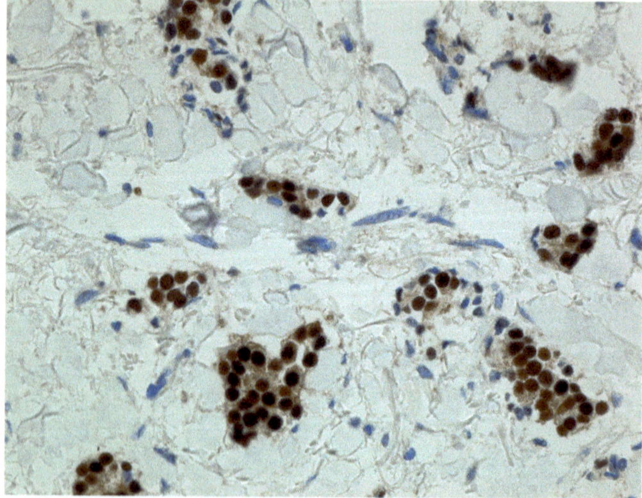

FIGURE 6.12 ER staining in well fixed tissue. In well-preserved tumor cells, ER signal is crisp and easy to assess. In fact, in this example, a faint cytoplasmic staining is also present, which represents preservation of cytoplasmic ER protein.

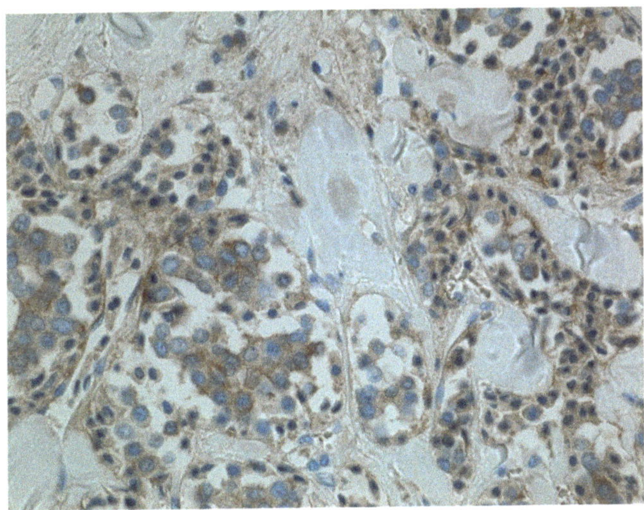

FIGURE 6.13 Early changes in HER2 protein due to suboptimal fixation. In this minimally autolyzed breast tumor, HER2 loss is already apparent. The staining is mainly in cytoplasm with rare cells showing weak membrane signal.

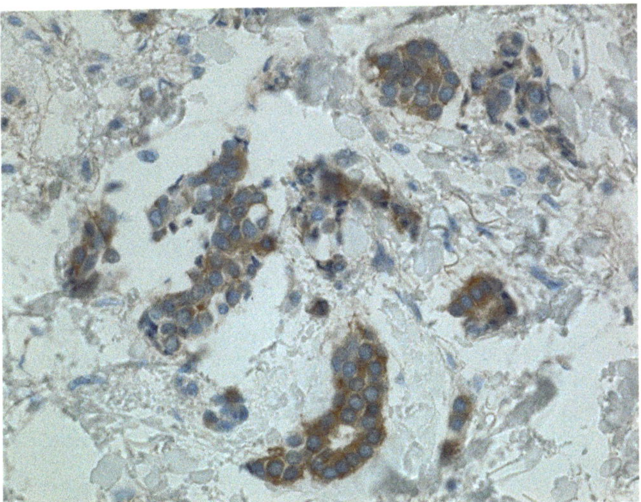

FIGURE 6.14 Complete loss of HER2 protein signal in a poorly fixed tumor. In an advanced stage of tissue loss, the alterations in molecular markers, such as HER2 are worse than morphologic changes. Here, the tumor cells can be recognized but HER2 membrane signal is lost leaving a light brown cytoplasmic blush.

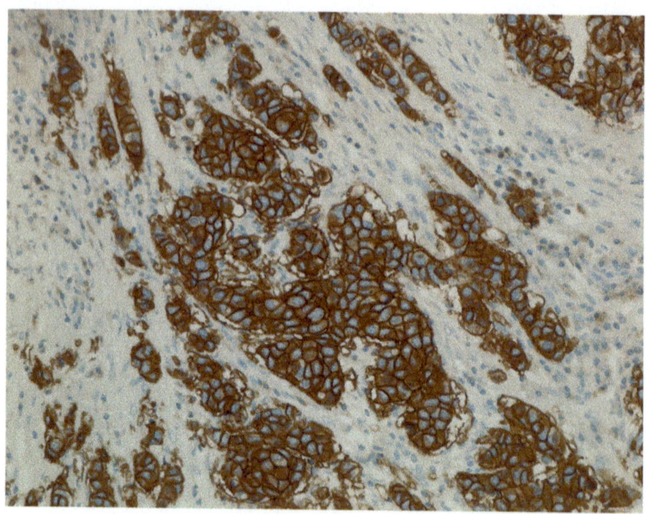

FIGURE 6.15 An example of positive HER2 staining in well-fixed tumor. In comparison to Figs. 6.13 and 6.14, the invasive ductal carcinoma in this case shows crisp membrane staining. Note the nuclei are negative and stain clearly with the counterstain.

TABLE 6.2 Effects of improper tissue preservation on assessment of predictive biomarkers.

- Both the proteins and nucleic acids are highly susceptible to delayed or inadequate tissue fixation.
- Membrane bound proteins, such as HER2 can be lost fairly early in case of delayed fixation and can result in a false-negative result.
- Nuclear bound proteins, particularly ER has been shown to be affected and appear as false negative in both under and over-fixed tissues.
- Underfixation in formalin can lead to false-positive biomarker result due to predominant tissue fixation in alcohol-based solutions, when the standardized assays optimized for optimal formalin fixation are employed.
- Failure to follow the tissue fixation guidelines can lead to erroneous or no results for biomarkers and can potentially lead to a need for new sample and thus poor patient care.

are optimized for adequately formalin-fixed tissue samples and the antigen retrieval conditions in the standardized assays may be too harsh for such under fixed tissues, giving nonspecific staining patterns (Table 6.2).

STANDARD OPERATING PROCEDURES (SOP) FOR HANDLING BREAST SPECIMENS

The development of SOP for breast specimens requires close communication and cooperation between the laboratory management and their counterparts in operating rooms, radiology suites, surgery centers, and doctor's offices. Since it is not possible to predict what types of breast specimen may contain malignancy, the only way to consistently acquire the collection time is to mandate the documentation of tissue collection date and time for all types of breast specimens, either on the specimen container or requisition or both. A laboratory may consider some exceptions to these standards, e.g., the specimen with extremely low probability of containing tumor, such as abscesses or re-excision of previously positive margins. Some of the steps that can help with the development of SOP covering extradepartmental activities affecting breast tissue handling are described in Table 6.3.

These standards have created workflow issues in all the laboratories handling such specimens. As the first step, the SOP for the gross room should define the time to fixation and fixation duration and its importance should be taught to all the staff. After proper education, these steps need to be considered during the development of SOP in the laboratory (Table 6.4).

The evaluation of standard characteristics of the tumor, such as tumor size, location, focality, margins, lymph nodes status, are requirements for accreditation of cancer programs by the CAP and the American College of Surgeons (ACOS) and required by the Commission on Cancer (CoC). The documentation for these required elements is completely dependent on accurate and thorough gross examination (Tables 6.5 and 6.6). With increased screening, there is a substantial increase in detection and then excision of nonpalpable lesions, including in situ and some invasive cancers. The gross examination and sectioning of breast specimens with such lesions is complex and time consuming. The method for assessing tumor size of nonpalpable lesions is described in Chap. 4. Several other aspects of the CAP tumor summary for invasive breast cancer and DCIS pertain to gross examination of the breast specimen. In order to consistently record these important pieces of information, the use of templates for gross examination is encouraged. Such templates not only improve consistency, but they can also help prevent repetition and unnecessary redundancy in breast pathology reports. This helps keep the report shorter, leads to less errors, and more importantly makes these reports easy to read. An example of gross description of a breast specimen using a template is provided in Table 6.7.

TABLE 6.3 Steps needed to implement handling of breast specimens prior to reaching the gross room.

- Inform the hospital committees about the new requirements. These include but are not limited to the operating room committee, cancer committee, patient safety, and quality committee and surgery center and physician's office staff.
- Consider at least an annual educational in-service for staff in various departments, where breast specimens are collected.
- Redesign of specimen submission form to provide highlighted fields for documenting date and time of specimen collection.
- In the institutions where the specimen requisition is created electronically, one needs to modify the required fields to include the date and time of collection.
- For core needle biopsies, the tumor is at the surface and tissue fixation begins immediately; therefore, the cold ischemia time in radiology and office suites is typically very short and high degree of compliance is easily achieved.
- The compliance data should be collected by the gross room supervisor or manager and periodically shared with the staff outside the department for feedback.
- In institutions with training programs, the orientation package and presentation to the new trainees should include emphasis on these requirements.
- The education of surgeons and radiologists is equally important, so they can serve as a reminder to their staff, who typically complete the specimen labeling and associated paperwork.
- For places without a pathologist on site and in busy centers, one should consider use of sterile specimen inking kit by the surgeon to mark the surfaces.
- Inking by the surgeon has two potential advantages: (1) this ensures accurate specimen orientation and (2) in certain situations it becomes safe to ask the surgeon to make a few slices through the tumor after inking the margins and place the specimen with some surgical gauze in a large formalin container.
- In order to meet these standards, the turnaround time for pathology report is often affected; thus patient education materials and postprocedure care instructions given to the patient, should mention these requirements.
- These steps help set the appropriate expectations and also reassure the patients that their tissue sample is being handled according to the standards.

TABLE 6.4 Steps needed to develop SOP in the gross room to handle breast specimens.

- The larger breast specimens, such as lumpectomy, needle localization, and mastectomy, are at risk for prolonged cold ischemia time. It is best to consider them as high-priority specimens, such as frozen section cases. This helps establish a system for rapid transport from the operating room or surgery center to the gross room.
- The gross room staff or the pathologist should attend to these specimens immediately to ink and then slice the tissue to expose the tumor. At this time, tissue can be exposed to formalin for fixation either by immediate sectioning or fixation and grossing later. In the latter case, one must ensure that tumor is in direct contact with large amounts of fresh formalin (the ideal ratio is 1:20).
- In situations where the surgical breast specimens are transported to a central location for grossing, the steps mentioned above should be accomplished at the site where the specimen is obtained, prior to transportation.
- The hours of the day the gross room is staffed may need to be adjusted based on each laboratory's needs.
- Establish tissue-processing times for breast samples to ensure that the tissue fixation duration falls between 6 and 48 or 72 h. Care should be taken for the last working day before long weekends and holidays.
- This leads to defining cut-off times for specimen grossing and subsequent processing. These cut-off times should be clearly communicated to the radiologists and the surgeons. They should be encouraged to discuss this with the patient.
- Use of templates for the dictation helps as a reminder to dictate/record the tissue collection date and time, fixation start and end times. The actual fixation duration can then be calculated and recorded in the final pathology report.
- The procedure manual for immunohistochemistry/in situ hybridization for ER, PR, and HER2 should reference these procedures.

TABLE 6.5 Required elements of gross examination for the CAP invasive breast cancer summary.

- Specimen
- Procedure
- Lymph node sampling
- Specimen integrity
- Specimen size
- Specimen laterality
- Tumor site (quadrant or o'clock position)
- Tumor focality
- Tumor size
- Presence of nipple, skin, and muscle

Table 6.6 Required elements of gross examination for the CAP DCIS summary.

- Specimen/procedure
- Specimen integrity
- Specimen size
- Lymph node sampling
- Specimen laterality
- Tumor site (quadrant)
- Topography of lesion and sections (to estimate the extent of DCIS)

Table 6.7 A sample gross description of a lumpectomy specimen using a template.

Specimen laterality: Right breast

Surgical procedure: Lumpectomy with wire localization

Measurements and weight: 3.2 cm (anterior–posterior) × 6.5 cm (superior–inferior) × 7.2 cm (medial–lateral); 75 g

Inking protocol: Anterior – orange; posterior – black; superior – purple; inferior – green; medial – blue; lateral – yellow

Tumor description: Located in the medial half of the specimen. It is gray and firm with irregular borders and retracted cut-surface. It measures 2.8 × 2.2 × 1.5 cm. The nearest margin is medial at 4 mm; all other margins are more than 10 mm.

Additional findings: Biopsy cavity 1.0 × 0.8 cm in the center of the tumor. No other lesions.

Cassette summary: A1 – tumor with medial margin; A2–4 – tumor with superior, anterior and posterior margins; A5 – inferior margin; A6 – tumor in relation to the biopsy cavity; A7–9 – uninvolved breast tissue; A10 – lateral margin (please see attached diagram also).

Suggested Reading

Anscher MS, Jones P, Prosnitz LR, et al. Local failure and margin status in early-stage breast carcinoma treated with conservation surgery and radiation therapy. Ann Surg. 218(1):22–8.1993.

Arora N, Martins D, Huston TL, et al. Sentinel node positivity rates with and without frozen section for breast cancer. Ann Surg Oncol. 15(1):256–61.2008.

Arriagada R, Le MG, Rochard F, et al. Conservative treatment versus mastectomy in early breast cancer: patterns of failure with 15 years of follow-up data. Institut Gustave-Roussy Breast Cancer Group. J Clin Oncol. 14(5):1558–64.1996.

Barranger E, Antoine M, Grahek D, et al. Intraoperative imprint cytology of sentinel nodes in breast cancer. J Surg Oncol. 86(3):128–33.2004.

Blumencranz P, Whitworth PW, Deck K, et al. Scientific Impact Recognition Award. Sentinel node staging for breast cancer: intraoperative molecular pathology overcomes conventional histologic sampling errors. Am J Surg. 194(4):426–32.2007.

Borger J, Kemperman H, Hart A, et al. Risk factors in breast-conservation therapy. J Clin Oncol. 12(4):653–60.1994.

Cabioglu N, Hunt KK, Sahin AA, et al. Role for intraoperative margin assessment in patients undergoing breast-conserving surgery. Ann Surg Oncol. 14(4):1458–71.2007.

Chagpar A, Yen T, Sahin A, et al. Intraoperative margin assessment reduces reexcision rates in patients with ductal carcinoma in situ treated with breast-conserving surgery. Am J Surg. 186(4):371–7.2003.

Chan SW, LaVigne KA, Port ER, et al. Does the benefit of sentinel node frozen section vary between patients with invasive duct, invasive lobular, and favorable histologic subtypes of breast cancer? Ann Surg. 247(1):143–9.2008.

S.K. Mohsin, *Frozen Section Library: Breast*, Frozen Section Library 9,
DOI 10.1007/978-1-4614-0718-8,

Contractor K, Gohel M, Al-Salami E, et al. Intra-operative imprint cytology for assessing the sentinel node in breast cancer: results of its routine use over 8 years. Eur J Surg Oncol. 35(1):16–20.2009.

Cox C, Centeno B, Dickson D, et al. Accuracy of intraoperative imprint cytology for sentinel lymph node evaluation in the treatment of breast carcinoma. Cancer. 105(1):13–20.2005.

Cox CE, Ku NN, Reintgen DS, et al. Touch preparation cytology of breast lumpectomy margins with histologic correlation. Arch Surg. 126(4):490–3.1991.

Cox CE, Pendas S, Ku NN, et al. Local recurrence of breast cancer after cytological evaluation of lumpectomy margins. Am Surg. 64(6):533–7; discussion 7–8.1998.

Creager AJ, Geisinger KR, Shiver SA, et al. Intraoperative evaluation of sentinel lymph nodes for metastatic breast carcinoma by imprint cytology. Mod Pathol. 15(11):1140–7.2002.

Cutress RI, McDowell A, Gabriel FG, et al. Observational and cost analysis of the implementation of breast cancer sentinel node intraoperative molecular diagnosis. J Clin Pathol. 63(6):522–9.2010.

D'Halluin F, Tas P, Rouquette S, et al. Intra-operative touch preparation cytology following lumpectomy for breast cancer: a series of 400 procedures. Breast. 18(4):248–53.2009.

Dewar JA, Arriagada R, Benhamou S, et al. Local relapse and contralateral tumor rates in patients with breast cancer treated with conservative surgery and radiotherapy (Institut Gustave Roussy 1970–1982). IGR Breast Cancer Group. Cancer. 76(11):2260–5.1995.

Edge SB, Byrd DR, Compton CC, et al. Breast. In: Edge SB, Byrd DR, Compton CC, et al., editors. AJCC Cancer Staging Manual. New York: 2010. p. 345–69, Springer.

Fisher B, Anderson S, Bryant J, et al. Twenty-year follow-up of a randomized trial comparing total mastectomy, lumpectomy, and lumpectomy plus irradiation for the treatment of invasive breast cancer. N Engl J Med. 347(16):1233–41.2002.

Fisher B, Montague E, Redmond C, et al. Findings from NSABP Protocol No. B-04-comparison of radical mastectomy with alternative treatments for primary breast cancer. I. Radiation compliance and its relation to treatment outcome. Cancer. 46(1):1–13.1980.

Fisher ER, Anderson S, Redmond C, et al. Pathologic findings from the National Surgical Adjuvant Breast Project protocol B-06. 10-year pathologic and clinical prognostic discriminants. Cancer. 71(8):2507–14.1993.

Fitzgibbons PL, LiVolsi VA. Recommendations for handling radioactive specimens obtained by sentinel lymphadenectomy. Surgical Pathology Committee of the College of American Pathologists, and the Association of Directors of Anatomic and Surgical Pathology. Am J Surg Pathol. 24(11):1549–51.2000.

Freedman G, Fowble B, Hanlon A, et al. Patients with early stage invasive cancer with close or positive margins treated with conservative surgery and radiation have an increased risk of breast recurrence that is delayed by adjuvant systemic therapy. Int J Radiat Oncol Biol Phys. 44(5):1005–15.1999.

Gemignani ML, Cody HS, 3rd, Fey JV, et al. Impact of sentinel lymph node mapping on relative charges in patients with early-stage breast cancer. Ann Surg Oncol. 7(8):575–80.2000.

Giuliano AE, Hunt KK, Ballman KV, et al. Axillary dissection vs no axillary dissection in women with invasive breast cancer and sentinel node metastasis: a randomized clinical trial. JAMA. 305(6):569–75.2011.

Hammond ME, Hayes DF, Dowsett M, et al. American Society of Clinical Oncology/College of American Pathologists guideline recommendations for immunohistochemical testing of estrogen and progesterone receptors in breast cancer. Arch Pathol Lab Med. 134(6):907–22.2010.

Henry-Tillman RS, Korourian S, Rubio IT, et al. Intraoperative touch preparation for sentinel lymph node biopsy: a 4-year experience. Ann Surg Oncol. 9(4):333–9.2002.

Holli K, Saaristo R, Isola J, et al. Lumpectomy with or without postoperative radiotherapy for breast cancer with favourable prognostic features: results of a randomized study. Br J Cancer. 84(2):164–9.2001.

Horvath JW, Barnett GE, Jimenez RE, et al. Comparison of intraoperative frozen section analysis for sentinel lymph node biopsy during breast cancer surgery for invasive lobular carcinoma and invasive ductal carcinoma. World J Surg Oncol. 7:34.2009.

Klimberg VS, Westbrook KC, Korourian S. Use of touch preps for diagnosis and evaluation of surgical margins in breast cancer. Ann Surg Oncol. 5(3):220–6.1998.

Komenaka IK, Torabi R, Nair G, et al. Intraoperative touch imprint and frozen section analysis of sentinel lymph nodes after neoadjuvant chemotherapy for breast cancer. Ann Surg. 251(2): 319–22.2010.

Langer I, Guller U, Berclaz G, et al. Accuracy of frozen section of sentinel lymph nodes: a prospective analysis of 659 breast cancer patients of the Swiss multicenter study. Breast Cancer Res Treat. 113(1):129–36.2009.

Layfield DM, Agrawal A, Roche H, et al. Intraoperative assessment of sentinel lymph nodes in breast cancer. Br J Surg. 98(1):4–17.2011.

Leidenius MH, Krogerus LA, Toivonen TS, et al. The feasibility of intraoperative diagnosis of sentinel lymph node metastases in breast cancer. J Surg Oncol. 84(2):68–73.2003.

Lester SC, Bose S, Chen YY, et al. Protocol for the examination of specimens from patients with ductal carcinoma in situ of the breast. Arch Pathol Lab Med. 133(1):15–25.2009.

Liu LC, Lang JE, Lu Y, et al. Intraoperative frozen section analysis of sentinel lymph nodes in breast cancer patients: a meta-analysis and single-institution experience. Cancer. 117(2):250–8.2011.

Liu LH, Siziopikou KP, Gabram S, et al. Evaluation of axillary sentinel lymph node biopsy by immunohistochemistry and multilevel sectioning in patients with breast carcinoma. Arch Pathol Lab Med. 124(11):1670–3.2000.

McLaughlin SA, Ochoa-Frongia LM, Patil SM, et al. Influence of frozen-section analysis of sentinel lymph node and lumpectomy margin status on reoperation rates in patients undergoing breast-conservation therapy. J Am Coll Surg. 206(1):76–82.2008.

Miller B, Brownell MD. A cooling method to improve sectioning of fatty breast specimens. Lab Medicine. 39(8):467–9.2008.

Mitchell ML. Frozen section diagnosis for axillary sentinel lymph nodes: the first six years. Mod Pathol. 18(1):58–61.2005.

Obedian E, Haffty BG. Internal mammary nodal irradiation in conservatively-managed breast cancer patients: is there a benefit? Int J Radiat Oncol Biol Phys. 44(5):997–1003.1999.

Olson TP, Harter J, Munoz A, et al. Frozen section analysis for intraoperative margin assessment during breast-conserving surgery results in low rates of re-excision and local recurrence. Ann Surg Oncol. 14(10):2953–60.2007.

Peterson ME, Schultz DJ, Reynolds C, et al. Outcomes in breast cancer patients relative to margin status after treatment with breast-conserving surgery and radiation therapy: the University of Pennsylvania experience. Int J Radiat Oncol Biol Phys. 43(5):1029–35.1999.

Poggi MM, Danforth DN, Sciuto LC, et al. Eighteen-year results in the treatment of early breast carcinoma with mastectomy versus breast conservation therapy: the National Cancer Institute Randomized Trial. Cancer. 98(4):697–702.2003.

Reitsamer R, Peintinger F, Prokop E, et al. 200 Sentinel lymph node biopsies without axillary lymph node dissection – no axillary recurrences after a 3-year follow-up. Br J Cancer. 90(8):1551–4.2004.

Renshaw AA. Adequate histologic sampling of breast core needle biopsies. Arch Pathol Lab Med. 125(8):1055–7.2001.

Saarela AO, Paloneva TK, Rissanen TJ, et al. Determinants of positive histologic margins and residual tumor after lumpectomy for early breast cancer: a prospective study with special reference to touch preparation cytology. J Surg Oncol. 66(4):248–53. 1997.

Sauer T, Engh V, Holck AM, et al. Imprint cytology of sentinel lymph nodes in breast cancer. Experience with rapid, intra-operative diagnosis and primary screening by cytotechnologists. Acta Cytol. 47(5):768–73.2003.

Schem C, Maass N, Bauerschlag DO, et al. One-step nucleic acid amplification-a molecular method for the detection of lymph node metastases in breast cancer patients; results of the German study group. Virchows Arch. 454(2):203–10.2009.

Schnitt SJ, Wang HH. Histologic sampling of grossly benign breast biopsies. How much is enough? Am J Surg Pathol. 13(6):505–12.1989.

Schrenk P, Konstantiniuk P, Wolfl S, et al. Intraoperative frozen section examination of the sentinel lymph node in breast cancer. Rozhl Chir. 84(5):217–22.2005.

Smitt MC, Nowels KW, Zdeblick MJ, et al. The importance of the lumpectomy surgical margin status in long-term results of breast conservation. Cancer. 76(2):259–67.1995.

Tamaki Y, Akiyama F, Iwase T, et al. Molecular detection of lymph node metastases in breast cancer patients: results of a multicenter trial using the one-step nucleic acid amplification assay. Clin Cancer Res. 15(8):2879–84.2009.

Taras AR, Hendrickson NA, Pugliese MS, et al. Intraoperative evaluation of sentinel lymph nodes in invasive lobular carcinoma of the breast. Am J Surg. 197(5):643–6; discussion 6–7.2009.

Teng S, Dupont E, McCann C, et al. Do cytokeratin-positive-only sentinel lymph nodes warrant complete axillary lymph node dissection in patients with invasive breast cancer? Am Surg. 66(6):574–8.2000.

Tew K, Irwig L, Matthews A, et al. Meta-analysis of sentinel node imprint cytology in breast cancer. Br J Surg. 92(9):1068–80.2005.

Turner RR, Hansen NM, Stern SL, et al. Intraoperative examination of the sentinel lymph node for breast carcinoma staging. Am J Clin Pathol. 112(5):627–34.1999.

Valdes EK, Boolbol SK, Ali I, et al. Intraoperative touch preparation cytology for margin assessment in breast-conservation surgery: does it work for lobular carcinoma? Ann Surg Oncol. 14(10):2940–5.2007.

van de Vrande S, Meijer J, Rijnders A, et al. The value of intraoperative frozen section examination of sentinel lymph nodes in breast cancer. Eur J Surg Oncol. 35(3):276–80.2009.

van Dongen JA, Voogd AC, Fentiman IS, et al. Long-term results of a randomized trial comparing breast-conserving therapy with mastectomy: European Organization for Research and Treatment of Cancer 10801 trial. J Natl Cancer Inst. 92(14):1143–50.2000.

Veronesi U, Paganelli G, Galimberti V, et al. Sentinel-node biopsy to avoid axillary dissection in breast cancer with clinically negative lymph-nodes. Lancet. 349(9069):1864–7.1997.

Veys I, Majjaj S, Salgado R, et al. Evaluation of the histological size of the sentinel lymph node metastases using RT-PCR assay: a rapid tool to estimate the risk of non-sentinel lymph node invasion in patients with breast cancer. Breast Cancer Res Treat. 124(3):599–605.2010.

Viale G, Dell'Orto P, Biasi MO, et al. Comparative evaluation of an extensive histopathologic examination and a real-time reverse-transcription-polymerase chain reaction assay for mammaglobin and cytokeratin 19 on axillary sentinel lymph nodes of breast carcinoma patients. Ann Surg. 247(1):136–42.2008.

Visser M, Jiwa M, Horstman A, et al. Intra-operative rapid diagnostic method based on CK19 mRNA expression for the detection of lymph node metastases in breast cancer. Int J Cancer. 122(11):2562–7.2008.

Wada N, Imoto S, Hasebe T, et al. Evaluation of intraoperative frozen section diagnosis of sentinel lymph nodes in breast cancer. Jpn J Clin Oncol. 34(3):113–7.2004.

Wazer DE, Schmidt-Ullrich RK, Ruthazer R, et al. Factors determining outcome for breast-conserving irradiation with margin-directed dose escalation to the tumor bed. Int J Radiat Oncol Biol Phys. 40(4):851–8.1998.

Weaver DL. Pathology evaluation of sentinel lymph nodes in breast cancer: protocol recommendations and rationale. Mod Pathol. 23 Suppl 2:S26-32.2010.

Weber S, Storm FK, Stitt J, et al. The role of frozen section analysis of margins during breast conservation surgery. Cancer J Sci Am. 3(5):273–7.1997.

Weiser MR, Montgomery LL, Susnik B, et al. Is routine intraoperative frozen-section examination of sentinel lymph nodes in breast cancer worthwhile? Ann Surg Oncol. 7(9):651–5.2000.

Wolff AC, Hammond ME, Schwartz JN, et al. American Society of Clinical Oncology/College of American Pathologists guideline recommendations for human epidermal growth factor receptor 2 testing in breast cancer. Arch Pathol Lab Med. 131(1):18–43.2007.

Zgajnar J, Frkovic-Grazio S, Besic N, et al. Low sensitivity of the touch imprint cytology of the sentinel lymph node in breast cancer patients--results of a large series. J Surg Oncol. 85(2):82–6; discussion 7.2004.

Index

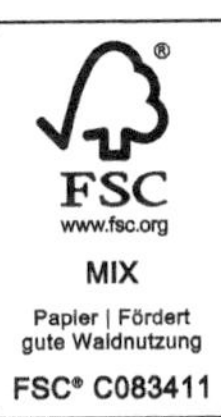

Zeitfracht Medien GmbH
Ferdinand-Jühlke-Straße 7
99095 Erfurt, Deutschland
produktsicherheit@kolibri360.de